The Wellness Blueprint

Rethink the Rules of Health
A Personalized Path to Fit Your Life
and Discover Your Full Potential

FREEMIND PRESS

CONTENTS

INTRODUCTION

It is late at night. Your phone's blue light is not the only thing keeping you awake. Concerned about your health, you scroll through a maze of wellness tips like eat this, avoid that, meditate, hydrate, run, rest. One headline claims that kale is a miracle. The next warns of hidden dangers in leafy greens. There are endless routines, miracle supplements, and secrets from influencers who promise a new you in thirty days or less. You want to feel better, stronger, and clearer. But the advice feels endless, even impossible. You close your phone and sigh, wondering if it is all just noise.

Just because you stop scrolling, it doesn't mean your mind stops racing. Perhaps it's overthinking and anxiety that impact your mental health. Maybe you wake up with a new ache every day. The rising prevalence of health conditions might mean you are suffering from a chronic disease. In 2020, 125 million Americans had at least one chronic condition, including hypertension, arthritis, respiratory diseases, cholesterol disorders, and chronic mental health conditions. In 2025, the figure is 164 million people, and this is estimated to reach 171 million in 2030 (American Hospital Association 2007). Whether you are trying to improve symptoms, lower the risk of chronic disorders, or hoping to lead a more fulfilling life, your wellness lies at the center.

However, like so many others, you may feel completely overwhelmed by the amount of health and wellness advice that is out there. And how do you know what is safe and backed by science rather than someone just trying to sell a product or get more followers? Maybe you have tried a new diet that left you hungry or tired. Maybe you bought a fitness gadget that now gathers dust. You may have followed morning routines that did not survive the first week. Most of us have faced disappointment. We have seen fads rise and fall. We have heard promises that sound too good to be true. Sometimes, it seems as if wellness is just another word for frustration.

This book exists because most modern health advice is more confusing than helpful. It is loud, scattered, and often based on hype rather than proof. Many plans expect you to fit your life into their mold. They do not see your late-night shifts, your busy family, or your unique body. They treat wellness like a one-size-fits-all t-shirt, never a perfect fit. This leads to guilt, confusion, and a sense that health is something far away. Let's face it, none of this is good for your confidence either.

But what if there was an alternative that allowed you to take control of your health? What if wellness was not about chasing trends, but about building something strong and lasting? What if you could design a life of health that fits who you are, where you live, and what you truly want?

This is the vision behind *The Wellness Blueprint*. We believe that true health is not a reaction to illness or a race toward perfection. Instead, it is a steady, personal pursuit. It draws on the best of modern science and ancient wisdom. It gives you the tools to shape your own path. You become the architect, building your health one choice at a time.

The Wellness Blueprint is committed to reshaping the concept of wellness into a practical reality accessible to everyone. It integrates practical wisdom, cutting-edge technology, and scientifically supported methods. This blueprint empowers you to reclaim control over your physical and mental wellness with confidence. It underscores the idea that health is not exclusive to professionals, celebrities, or individuals with ample leisure time. It's a universal right, belonging to you. We believe in sharing tools and knowledge that work in real life. They are simple, flexible, and built for busy adults, parents, shift workers, and anyone seeking change, no matter where they start.

This book does not offer a strict set of rules. You will not find a rigid program that punishes you for missing a day. Instead, you will discover a flexible "Wellness GPS." It helps you find your path, adjust your route, and celebrate progress. It adapts to your unique life, honors your individuality, and gives you science-backed steps you can trust.

Inside, you will build your own wellness plan. You will learn why your mindset matters and how to change it. You will discover how to eat in a way that nourishes, not restricts. You will find movement that energizes, not exhausts. You will discover ways to sleep better, manage stress, and build resilience. Above all, we will do this while appreciating the incredible connection between the body and mind. Each chapter gives you tools, checklists, and templates so you can put ideas into action right away. Real-world stories and tips show how others have found success on their own terms.

This book is guided by a new idea: "Wellness Wins." Here, success is not about ticking every box or reaching a magic number on the scale. It is about progress, resilience, and self-compassion. It is about how you feel, how you grow, and how you recover from setbacks. It is about celebrating small wins, even when the journey feels long.

At Freemind Press, we have faced a wide range of health challenges. We have fallen for the fleeting trends and discovered that something has to change. This was when *The Wellness Blueprint*, along with the Wellness GPS, was created. We did our homework, fact-checked, and put our findings into practice. Each time progress was felt, the passion to help others grew. We know that wellness is an individual thing, but that's not to say that we can't all be part of the same community.

As you turn the page, we encourage you to question old ideas and try something new. What if wellness was not a struggle, but a source of joy? What if you could design a life that supports your best self, every day? In the chapters ahead, we will rethink wellness for modern lives. We will explore what works, why it matters, and how you can make it your own.

Are you ready to start building your Wellness Blueprint? Let's find the beginning of your path and take one step at a time, together.

1

RETHINKING WELLNESS

A New Paradigm for Modern Lives

L et's clear something up straight away! If you have tried something in the past and didn't see the results you were hoping for, please don't listen to those who said you didn't try hard enough or that you didn't give it long enough. The issue wasn't and isn't laziness or lack of willpower. It's that these plans don't fit your actual life. Rigid meal plans don't survive a busy week, and fitness programs often require more time or equipment than you have. Trends that work for others leave you feeling like a failure when they don't work for you. The old model says, "Follow these steps and you'll succeed," but real life is unpredictable. Schedules shift, stress appears, and what worked for one person can fall apart in another's world. Wellness today is everywhere yet feels out of reach, as all the advice seems to contradict itself. This chapter offers a chance to step back from the chaos and discover what you need right now for the stage of life you are at.

THE WELLNESS GPS: PERSONALIZING YOUR PATH IN A NOISY WORLD

Think of wellness like a GPS: You set your destination, but the route adjusts for detours, traffic, or missed turns. It calmly recalculates, offering a new route with no judgment. Your wellness path should be just as adaptive and flexible. For example, a parent with three kids faces different challenges than a single remote worker. One may squeeze in exercise during school runs; the other may devote an uninterrupted hour to a walk. Both approaches are valid and worthy of respect.

Rigid plans rarely work because life is unpredictable. Adaptability is essential. If you skip a workout because your child is sick or you're tied up in meetings, that's just a detour, certainly not a failure. Your map still works; it just shifts as your circumstances do.

To build a personalized wellness plan, start by reflecting on your present reality, not with self-judgment but with honesty.

Where Are You Now? Self-Assessment Exercise

Jot down quick answers to these:

- Most mornings, do you feel energized or exhausted?
- Is your routine predictable or hectic?
- Are you moving your body as much as you'd like?
- What feels good in your health right now? What feels stuck?
- What recurring obstacle gets in your way?
- What aspects of your health are you pleased with?

Common places to start are burnout from stress, overwhelm from too many choices, or frustration at progress stalling. Every starting point is valid. It's simply your launchpad.

Comparison is another trap. Social media is full of unrealistic images of people who have achieved the perfect body in twenty-eight days. Again, we aren't saying that this isn't possible, but you don't see the challenges they face or the effort they put in. Research shows that comparing yourself to friends or influencers can hurt your motivation and self-esteem. It can add to poor body image, decrease overall well-being, and increase depression. Before you compare yourself to others on social media, remind yourself that many of these images have been heavily edited or are just fake (The Jed Foundation, n.d.). The messy middle, where growth happens, is rarely shown.

A friend once followed a fitness influencer religiously, investing in all the gear and mimicking every workout. When her results didn't match the online posts, she felt defeated and quit. She hadn't failed. She had simply set her GPS to someone else's coordinates.

You deserve to set your own wellness coordinates, the goals and milestones that are meaningful to you. Whether that means more energy for evening playtime with your kids, steadier moods, or simply moving consistently for ten minutes a day, your goals should serve your life.

Allow yourself to define success in personal ways: better sleep, staying patient under stress, or consistent movement. These are authentic wins that directly improve daily life. Your internal Wellness GPS will help you recalibrate through life's ups and downs and celebrate every forward step, no matter how modest.

Reflection Exercise

Grab yourself a new journal, notebook, or open a notes app (because you will need it throughout the chapters) and finish these prompts:

- My biggest challenge right now is ...
- I feel most energized when ...
- If I could achieve one thing this month, it would be ...

No single starting point is perfect, but there is always a path forward from wherever you are right now.

SCIENCE VS. HYPE: HOW TO TRUST WHAT REALLY WORKS

If you've ever been tempted by a "miracle" fat-burning tea or a new app that claims it will change everything with a seven-minute workout, you're not alone. The wellness world is buzzing with bold claims, but not all advice is created equal. It's easy to get swept up in hype, especially when you're tired, frustrated, or searching for a quick fix. These trends thrive on big promises: instant results, dramatic before-and-after pictures, and testimonials that sound too good to be true. The truth is, most of these fads don't stand up to real scrutiny. They prey on your hope and your desire for change. A classic red flag is any product or plan guaranteeing unbelievable results with minimal effort or sacrifice. If someone says you'll lose twenty pounds in two weeks, reverse aging overnight, or never feel anxious again just by taking a supplement or cutting out an entire food group, that's hype, plain and simple.

Take the example of the low-carb diet that sweeps across our social media pages, where people are encouraged to consume 70 to 80 percent of calories from fat. The problem with overly restrictive diets is that people end up missing whole food groups. As a result, people could end up with vitamin and mineral deficiencies. The low-carb diet has been linked to a higher risk for kidney issues, digestive problems, and possibly even an increased risk of heart disease (Coleman Collins 2025). This is why wellness trends need to be analyzed objectively.

You might wonder how to separate real science from the noise. A good place to start is to look for references and transparency. Reliable health advice is almost never based on one single study or an influencer's personal story; instead, it's grounded in peer-reviewed science and acknowledges both benefits and limitations. Sources like the Mayo Clinic, Cleveland Clinic, and Harvard Health Publishing are reliable (The Healthy League, n.d.). You will notice that they don't just highlight success. They explain risks and openly discuss where knowledge is evolving. You want to see recommendations that include citations from medical journals and clear explanations of how conclusions were reached. If a source can't tell you where its information comes from, or if it ignores the complexity and nuance of health, it's probably not worth your trust. For this reason, you will notice that all the science we cover is backed with in-text citations, where the information was found and the date it was published (or n.d. for no date). All these citations are listed in the reference section of this book, so you can visit the resource and discover more.

Uncertainty will always exist. Science is a process of discovery, not a list of final answers. Advice shifts over time. Remember in the early '80s when all fats were considered bad? We were encouraged to drink low-fat milk and avoid cheese and butter by doctors, the media, and government policies, but with little evidence to support this. Ironically, this was around the same time that the obesity pandemic began (Hinchman 2019). New research sometimes reverses old recommendations. That doesn't mean past advice was wrong on purpose. As technology evolves, we learn and adapt as better information becomes available. It's normal for your own approach to change, too, as you learn more about your body and what works for you.

It's actually a strength, not a weakness, to admit you don't have all the answers right away. Flexibility allows you to stay open to new evidence without feeling like you failed if your routine changes. It's healthy to experiment within reason and to keep what supports your well-being while letting go of what doesn't serve you anymore.

You don't have to become a medical expert to make sound choices about wellness. You do need to become a curious consumer—one who asks questions, seeks out reputable sources, and trusts that slow progress built on solid ground beats bold claims every single time.

Mythbusting Quick Reference

You don't need to spend hours investigating everything that appeals to you, but you should take a moment to look at the pros and the potential cons. When you run into new advice or products, whether it's an Instagram post pushing green juice cleanses or a coworker's favorite biohacking gadget, ask yourself a few key questions:

- What's the actual evidence? Does the claim cite research from credible journals or organizations?
- Who benefits financially if I believe or buy into this?
- Are both benefits and risks explained clearly?
- Does the recommendation work for many types of people, or only in ideal situations?
- Does it sound too good to be true?

If the answers leave you uneasy or the details are vague, pause before investing your time, energy, or money. If something feels off or too perfect, listen to that nudge of skepticism. The goal isn't to find the one perfect answer but to build habits on a foundation that lasts longer than any passing trend.

PROGRESS, NOT PERFECTION: REDEFINING SUCCESS AND SELF-COMPASSION

It's easy to think a single slip ruins your progress. Maybe you stuck to a new habit, then missed a workout, had a busy week, or indulged a little extra, and suddenly it feels like all your hard work is lost. This all-or-nothing thinking, fueled by perfectionism, makes people believe that if they can't do everything right, they should quit altogether. For some, one missed Monday becomes a skipped week, and soon, sneakers are gathering dust. Others take a more flexible approach, such as walking on Tuesday or doing some stretching at home instead, to keep moving forward. Research confirms this: People who focus on consistent, small steps are more likely to sustain habits than those striving for perfect streaks (Pattison Professional Counseling and Mediation Center, n.d.). Small efforts add up more than big but unsustainable gestures. Self-compassion is vital here. Interestingly, self-compassion is another area of life that has evolved. In the past, it was more common to be hard on ourselves as a way to push to achieve more and succeed. It's a competitive mentality, and why a degree of competition is motivating. When we compete against others, it impacts our self-worth. Let's imagine Jane and Fred started a new workout at the same time. Jane sees amazing results, but Fred feels like his progress is slow. Fred feels insecure and less worthy.

We have all been there, and probably more than once. You are on a good streak, and you slip. Maybe it's that donut that is staring at you, wanting to be eaten, or the takeout because you are too exhausted to cook. In the moment, it's a pleasure, but that soon becomes a guilty pleasure. Instead of criticizing yourself after a missed workout or unhealthy meal, speak to yourself as you would to a friend. If your friend felt bad for eating chips after a rough day, you'd likely reassure them: "Be kind to yourself; tomorrow is a new day." Offer that same kindness to yourself. This is the essence of self-compassion (Seppala 2014). When guilt or shame appear, try, "Today was tough, and my choices weren't ideal, but that doesn't erase my progress or worth. Off days are allowed." Self-compassion isn't about making excuses. It's about accepting that perfection doesn't exist, but doing your best does.

Curiosity helps, too. Rather than labeling yourself as bad, try to understand what led to the setback. Were you stressed, tired, or overwhelmed? Recognizing your triggers prepares you for next time. A trigger is any person, thing, place, or situation that causes you to react intensely or in an unexpected way. They are often related to past experiences, and you may notice physical responses like a racing heart or shortness of breath before you fully recognize what is happening. Your senses (like smelling Grandma's perfume after she passed away) are common triggers. Past trauma is another potential trigger (The University of North Carolina Chapel Hill, n.d.). Imagine if you are in a new spinning class and can't quite keep up, despite enjoying it. But you look to the next person and see them doing well, and you are flooded with memories of a parent or coach telling you that second place isn't good enough. Instead of letting those memories take over, go back to the question, "What would I tell a friend right now?" or alternatively, "What do I need to feel supported?" This shift from judgment to curiosity breaks perfectionism's grip and creates room for growth.

Redefine what wellness success looks like. The scale or mirror might give feedback, but they don't tell the whole story. Instead, notice how you feel when you wake up, how well you slept, if your mood stayed stable under stress, or if you moved your body more than before. These are true indicators of progress. Celebrate wins like improved sleep, steadier moods, more patience with family, or simply returning to your routine after a setback.

Sample Wellness Wins Log

Imagine a jar, or better yet, make one. Each time you see a small positive change, like fewer headaches, more energy, or a calm response to stress, write it on paper and drop it in the jar. Don't worry, you will soon have the tools to do all these things. Over time, these notes show your steady progress.

Consistency and tracking small wins help maintain motivation and remind you that meaningful change is happening, even if it feels slow. Setbacks are inevitable, but they don't erase your gains. Instead of spiraling into guilt, recalibrate with this quick routine:

1. **Breathe:** Take a pause and notice what happened, without self-judgment.
2. **Reflect:** Consider what got in the way—stress, schedule conflicts, or unexpected events?
3. **Reset:** Pick one small thing you can do today, like drinking more water or walking for five minutes.
4. **Re-engage:** Show up again tomorrow, no matter how imperfectly.

Growth isn't about perfect weeks or never making mistakes. It's about continually picking yourself back up. Some days it will be easier, others harder. Lasting wellness depends on self-compassion and persistence every day. The path will have bumps and restarts, and they are normal and necessary parts of real change. Every time you're kind to yourself after a setback, you build strength to continue.

Here is a mantra to start each day: Celebrate every win, even small ones. Take this one step further and consider if it's the smaller ones that matter more, because they are what gives you momentum. Letting go of perfectionism and embracing self-compassion are essential components of a growth mindset. So, let's jump straight into the next chapter and find out what it takes to master the growth mindset.

2

MINDSET FIRST

The Foundation of Lasting Wellness

W hen you try something new and it doesn't work out, it's easy to conclude, "I'm just not the kind of person who does this." But your mindset is quietly shaping that belief. Before we explore what the growth mindset is, we are going to take a fascinating trip deep into the brain and its inner workings. It's time to dissect the thought process!

HOW YOUR MINDSET IS SHAPED

Okay, this is going to require a little science, but we promise it will be worth it. After this section, there will be no more telling yourself that you can't do something or that you can't teach an old dog new tricks. Welcome to the world of neuroplasticity!

Neuroplasticity refers to the brain's remarkable ability to reorganize and adapt throughout life. Contrary to older beliefs that the brain's structure was fixed after a certain age, neuroscience has shown that the brain is constantly changing in response to experiences, learning, and even thoughts. The brain has approximately eighty-six billion neurons, and each experience we have causes neurons to connect to another, known as a synapse or neural pathway. Your brain contains around 100 trillion neuropathways, and none of them are fixed. The neural pathways in our brain can strengthen, weaken, form new connections, or even fade away (Caruso 2023). Whether you're learning a new language, recovering from injury, or working to shift negative thought patterns, your brain is always reshaping itself.

When we experience thoughts and emotions, the brain processes them through networks involving different regions, like the prefrontal cortex (for reasoning and decision-making), the amygdala (for emotional responses), and the hippocampus (for memory) (Cleveland Clinic 2024a). The more you repeat a negative thought about yourself, such as self-criticism or feelings of worthlessness, the stronger the neural pathway becomes, and the easier it is to remember. The more we think about them, the more the brain "wires" those patterns as habits (Cherry 2024b).

Let's look at a practical example of neuroplasticity. Imagine you want to take up salsa dancing. At first, you have two left feet because the neurons have only just fired together. But each time you repeat the steps, it gets easier because the neurons have wired together. Nevertheless, if you don't practice for a few weeks, you notice the steps are more challenging to remember. And if you stop practicing altogether, the neural pathways break, a process known as synaptic pruning (Cherry 2024b).

In short, while our brains may hold on to patterns, especially negative ones, out of habit or conditioning, they are also capable of growth and transformation. By being intentional with our thoughts and behaviors, we can literally shape our brains to support greater mental health and self-worth.

THE FIXED VS. GROWTH MINDSET

The concept of a growth mindset, developed by Carol Dweck, is a theory that can greatly alter your approach to wellness. A growth mindset is the belief that your abilities, habits, and health can improve with effort, learning, and smart strategies. In contrast, a fixed mindset assumes you're stuck with your current skills (Maguire 2024). Instead of boxing yourself in with "I'm not a runner," or "I can't cook healthy meals," you start thinking, "I'm learning to move more," or "I'm figuring out healthy cooking." This shift, though subtle, opens up options you may have overlooked.

Research shows that a fixed mindset is linked to setting performance-based goals, believing abilities are unchangeable when facing failure, and responding to challenges with helpless behavior, whereas the growth mindset shows that people are more likely to thrive when facing challenges and continue to improve (Yeager & Dweck 2020). Now that you understand neuroplasticity, you can see that the growth mindset is possible, and you can improve your skills and abilities. In wellness, the fixed mindset shows up as giving up after one attempt at yoga or assuming you'll never like vegetables because you didn't as a kid. Imagine trying meal prep for the first time because a friend inspired you on Instagram. The fixed mindset chimes in: "You're just not organized; meal prep isn't for you." But with a growth mindset, you think, "This week didn't go as planned. What can I tweak? Maybe fewer meals at once, or new recipes next time." That willingness to experiment paves the way for progress.

The same logic applies to learning a breathing exercise for stress relief. The first time feels awkward, maybe you get distracted or feel silly at your desk. A fixed mindset says, "I'm just not good at this." Growth mindset thinking says, "New things always feel awkward at first. The more I practice, the easier it gets." This subtle difference is critical. Those who believe they can improve are more likely to try again after setbacks and are less harsh on themselves. Importantly, a growth mindset doesn't mean pretending everything is easy. It means seeing obstacles as part of the process, not proof you're bound to fail.

So, how do you build this mindset into daily life? Start by noticing your inner dialogue and gently shifting it. Try reflection prompts like, "What did I learn from today's challenge?" instead of just, "Did I succeed?" In Dweck's TED Talk, she explains the power of yet. By simply adding the word yet to the end of negative self-talk, you can change your mindset. Look at the difference between "I can't run five miles" to "I can't run five miles yet." The second sentence is a reminder that progress, though it takes time and effort, is possible (Farnam Street, n.d.).

Reflection Exercise: Mindset Reframe

Write down a wellness area where you feel stuck (nutrition, sleep, movement, etc.). List the thoughts that come up when things don't go as planned. Next to each, write a growth-minded alternative. For example:

- **Fixed:** "I always mess up my sleep schedule."
- **Growth:** "Sleep has been tough lately, but I can try new routines and see what helps."

This approach can be transformative. Mike, a friend of ours, felt anxious at the gym, worrying others judged his form. Initially, he skipped workouts if he felt insecure. Learning about a growth mindset, he started viewing each session as practice, telling himself, "Each workout teaches me about my body." Gradually, his anxiety lessened, and his confidence grew, not because he became perfect, but because he dropped that expectation.

Jasmine told us about how she slipped back into old eating habits after months of healthy cooking. Though disappointed, she didn't call it a failure. She asked what had changed and what she could adjust. When she switched her focus to learning rather than loss, Jasmine found motivation and actually enjoyed starting again.

Growth mindset isn't about forced positivity or ignoring real struggles. It's about seeing value in effort and finding lessons in every attempt. When you stop labeling yourself and see yourself as a work in progress, wellness becomes about continual discovery, not just checking boxes.

BREAKING THE ALL-OR-NOTHING TRAP: OVERCOMING PERFECTION PARALYSIS

All-or-nothing thinking sneaks into wellness routines like an unwelcome guest. You start the week excited, but then life throws a curveball. The old script plays in your mind: "I blew it. The whole week is ruined." Sound familiar? It's the classic black-and-white trap where either you're good or off the rails. This mind trick shows up everywhere: Eating a cookie means the diet is over; missing one night of good sleep means there's no use trying to improve; skipping meditation once means you might as well give up. The smallest detour can make you feel like you've failed completely, even when the reality is just a single off day. This type of cognitive disorder can lead to everything being perfect (all) or a failure (nothing) and a lack of appreciation for all the grays (Jones 2023).

This perfection-or-bust mindset is more than just a minor annoyance. The pressure to do everything right often leads to avoidance. If you can't do it perfectly, why bother trying at all? Research into perfectionism shows that people with strict, unforgiving standards are actually more likely to burn out. We aren't just talking about exhaustion and irritability. Symptoms of burnout include anxiety, depression, a lack of motivation, memory issues, and social withdrawal. Physical symptoms can include headaches and nausea (Kluger 2023). If you set the bar at 100 percent, never missing a workout, always eating clean, meditating every day, it doesn't take much to feel like you're falling short. It becomes more likely that you drop your healthy habits after only a few slip-ups, not because you lacked motivation, but because your standards were impossible to maintain.

The good news is, you can break this cycle with some practical strategies that make room for real life. One of the simplest tools is what we call minimum viable wellness. Instead of aiming for the perfect version of your goal, choose the tiniest version you can manage on hard days (Donovan, n.d.). Maybe your plan was a forty-five-minute workout, but your energy is gone after work. Give yourself permission to stretch for five minutes or walk around the block. This brings momentum back when things stall. Another favorite strategy is the "two-minute rule." If starting feels overwhelming, commit to just two minutes (Clear 2013). Tell yourself you'll only put on your sneakers and do a couple of jumping jacks, or just chop one vegetable for lunch prep. Often, getting started is enough to push through inertia, and if not, you've still kept your promise to yourself.

Building a resilience buffer is also powerful. Plan ahead for imperfect days by creating backup options, like having frozen veggies on hand for quick meals or keeping a yoga mat near your desk for ten-minute movement bursts. Micro-goals help here, too. Instead of aiming for perfection, focus on any improvement over doing nothing. If you usually skip self-care when tired, ask yourself, "What's one tiny thing I can do today?" It might be taking three deep breaths before bed or drinking an extra glass of water. Even these small acts add to your wellness.

These small wins deserve celebration. Partial successes aren't just better than nothing. They actually train your brain to notice effort and progress, which boosts motivation for next time. Celebrating your achievements activates the brain's reward system, releasing the feel-good hormone dopamine, which reinforces positive behaviors. The brain's reward system is also tied to increased resilience and less risk of burnout (CompassAI 2025). Try tracking any day you complete even the smallest healthy action. A simple chart on your fridge or in your notes app works wonders. Mark an X for any movement (walk, stretch, dance), mindful moment (deep breath, pause), or nutritious meal or snack. At the end of the week, count those marks and see how many times you showed up for yourself, even if imperfectly.

This reminded us of when we heard from a reader named Alex who wanted to run three times a week but struggled to keep up with a strict schedule. After missing a couple of runs, he almost gave up completely. Instead, he switched to celebrating every time he laced up his shoes, even if he only managed a ten-minute jog or a brisk walk around the block. Over time, those short efforts added up. When tracking any movement as a win, Alex built confidence and actually ended up running more often in the long run.

Progress isn't measured by perfect streaks. It's built on stringing together small steps and refusing to let one missed day erase everything. When you stop thinking in absolutes and start honoring every bit of effort, wellness becomes about persistence instead of perfection. That shift helps make routines sustainable, flexible, and much more forgiving, qualities that keep you coming back, no matter how many times life gets messy.

Try this: Next time you feel the urge to quit after one missed workout or meal, pause and ask yourself—what's one thing I can do right now that moves me in the direction I want to go? Then celebrate that action fully.

Over time, these small pivots chip away at all-or-nothing thinking and help you find real satisfaction in progress rather than flawless results.

SELF-COMPASSION SCRIPTS: TRANSFORMING GUILT AND SHAME INTO MOTIVATION

The discomfort of shame and guilt is actually damaging to your motivation. When you beat yourself up over missteps, you set off a cycle that makes it harder to try again. Harsh self-criticism eats away at hope and increases the chance you'll give up completely. It becomes a self-fulfilling prophecy where you tell yourself you are only going to end up making the same mistake, and inevitably, you do.

Here's where self-compassion scripts make a difference. Positive affirmations are short, powerful statements that individuals repeat to themselves to challenge and overcome negative thoughts or self-sabotaging beliefs. The science behind affirmations lies in their ability to engage the brain's reward system and promote neuroplasticity. MRI scans show that affirmations activate brain regions associated with self-processing and valuation, such as the ventromedial prefrontal cortex. This helps individuals internalize positive beliefs and reduce stress by shifting attention away from threats or self-doubt. Studies have shown that self-affirmation can enhance problem-solving abilities under pressure, improve self-esteem, and support behavior change (Moore 2019). While they're not a cure-all, positive affirmations can be a valuable psychological tool for a more optimistic mindset and promoting emotional resilience.

For positive affirmations to be effective, they have to have meaning to you. If you feel like an idiot when you are repeating them, your brain is hardly going to reward you with a dash of dopamine. Below are examples of affirmations related to physical and mental wellness, but feel free to tweak them for a more personal approach.

- My body is strong, capable, and supports me every day.
- I nourish my mind and body with kindness and respect.
- Every breath I take fills me with calm and clarity.
- I am worthy of rest, healing, and inner peace.

- I choose to focus on what I can control and let go of what I cannot.
- My mental health is just as important as my physical health.
- I am becoming healthier, stronger, and more balanced each day.
- It's okay to slow down and listen to what my body needs.
- I release self-judgment and welcome self-compassion.
- Healing is not linear, and I honor my progress every step of the way.

Developing a compassionate inner dialogue takes practice, but it's surprisingly simple once you have the right tools. One practical exercise is to grab a piece of paper or open your phone's notes app and jot down three negative thoughts you catch yourself thinking about wellness slip-ups. Maybe it's, "I failed again," or, "I always mess this up," or, "I'll never get it together." Once they're out of your head and onto the page, rewrite each one as if you were comforting a friend. For example, "I failed again" could become, "I'm learning what works for me, and every setback teaches me something." Or take, "I always mess this up," and turn it into, "I haven't got it right yet." Even tough weeks start to feel lighter when your self-talk shifts from criticism to understanding.

You can keep these rewritten phrases somewhere visible—on a sticky note by your mirror or as reminders on your phone. Repeating these scripts gives them more power as your neurons wire together. Over time, this new language becomes second nature. You might catch yourself starting with old criticism but quickly switching gears.

What's remarkable is how much self-compassion impacts actual results. One reader shared how she'd quit countless diets because the guilt after eating something off-plan felt overwhelming. Once she started using self-compassion scripts, reminding herself that one meal doesn't erase progress, she found it easier to get back on track without punishing herself. She also found it easier to forgive herself when slip-ups happened.

Self-forgiveness is not letting yourself off the hook. It is the compassionate process of accepting your mistakes without harsh self-judgment.

It involves recognizing that being human means being imperfect and understanding that errors are opportunities for growth, not permanent reflections of your worth (Luskin & Harris 2025). Rather than dwelling in guilt or shame, self-forgiveness allows you to learn from the experience, make amends if needed, and move forward with greater wisdom and kindness toward yourself. It's a vital part of emotional healing and building resilience.

Exercise: Rewriting Self-Talk

Find a quiet space, take a deep breath, and grab your journal. Set a timer for five minutes. Write freely, don't worry about grammar or structure. Let your thoughts flow without judgment. Follow the steps to practice self-forgiveness.

- **Step 1:** Recall a mistake or decision you still feel bad about. Briefly describe what happened. What were you feeling at the time? What was your intention?
- **Step 2:** Reflect on how you've grown since then. What have you learned from the experience? How has it shaped you or helped you become wiser, stronger, or more compassionate?
- **Step 3:** Write a statement of forgiveness to yourself. For example: "I forgive myself for …" or "I was doing the best I could with what I knew." Be honest and gentle.
- **Step 4:** End with an affirmation. For example: "I deserve peace," or "I am allowed to move on and grow."

To wrap up this chapter, remember that mindset matters as much as any meal plan or workout schedule. Growth and resilience start with how you treat yourself when things get messy. Progress thrives where kindness and self-compassion live. Next up, we'll explore how tiny habits, built from this foundation of understanding, lead to big changes over time.

3

HABIT SCIENCE

Micro-Changes for Maximum Impact

Imagine standing in your kitchen, waiting for your coffee to brew, going through motions on autopilot. Now, imagine using that instant to add something new, like a deep breath, a stretch, or jotting down gratitude. We are living in a fast-paced world, and it can feel like finding time to achieve your goals and make lasting change is almost impossible. If the thought of taking an hour or so out of your day to work on your wellness makes you feel guilty, this chapter is for you.

INCORPORATING HABITS INTO YOUR ROUTINE

Habit stacking is a practical method for making new habits stick by linking them to routines you already perform. Coined by James Clear, experts see habit stacking as a form of self-directed neuroplasticity (Cleveland Clinic 2024b). Think of daily habits as anchors, as solid, unchanging actions you do almost without thinking. By tying a new habit to one of these anchors, your brain starts treating both actions as a single unit, making it effortless to adopt the new behavior. You simply ride the flow of an existing routine, using its momentum to launch a new, small action.

The key is identifying your personal anchor habits. Observe what you already do naturally, things like sipping your favorite morning drink, walking your dog before work, brushing your teeth before bed, and sitting at your desk in the morning. These dependably recurring moments are prime spots for attaching new habits.

Anchor Habit Finder: Interactive Exercise

Take a notepad and list out everything you do on a typical weekday, from waking up to bedtime. Without filtering, just jot them down. These are your anchor habits, ideal foundations for introducing something new.

Here's how to build your first habit stack:

1. Pick one of your anchor habits, let's say brushing your teeth before bed.
2. Choose a simple action to tack on, something quick and easy like a two-minute stretch, a gratitude note, or a glass of water.
3. Each day, perform this new action immediately after your anchor habit. Keep a small tracker (an app, calendar, or sticky note) to mark your consistency.

The secret is consistency, not ambition. There's no need to overhaul your whole routine. "Stretch after brushing my teeth" is much easier to remember than just "stretch every night." The anchor leads the new habit.

Here are real-world examples:

- Five minutes of a brain training app after doing the dishes.
- Prepare your clothes for the next day after a shower.
- Ten push-ups between each video game level.
- Taking vitamins after brushing your teeth.
- Planning your day after meditating (Reddit, n.d.).

Habit stacking fits any lifestyle. If you travel for work, it might mean rolling your shoulders after buckling your airplane seat belt or taking a brief walk after every Zoom meeting. If your evenings vary but your mornings are routine, try setting a daily intention after your first coffee. The goal is to make the new action so closely tied to the anchor that omitting it feels abnormal.

People often overestimate what they can achieve in a week and underestimate what small actions compound into over months. Habit stacking lets your brain's circuitry take over through repeated, consistent pairing of behaviors. Tracking your progress reinforces your stack and provides a little mental reward each time you check it off, boosting your confidence and momentum.

If you're unsure where to start, revisit your Anchor Habit Finder. Choose just one anchor and a tiny new habit (no more than two minutes). Pair them until they merge seamlessly. Over time, these small changes will stick and pave the way for more positive shifts with minimal extra effort.

MICRO-GOALS AND MOMENTUM: DESIGNING TINY WINS THAT STICK

If you've ever felt overwhelmed by big health goals, whether it's training for a marathon, overhauling your diet, or meditating for an hour a day, you're not alone. The brain reacts to massive change with stress, making it much more likely for you to freeze up or put things off. There's real science behind this. When you set huge goals, your brain's alarm system can actually kick in, especially the amygdala, which is responsible for the body's stress response. It's the stress response that can make larger objectives seem overwhelming before you even begin (Thompson 2025). The solution is micro-goals. These are the smallest possible actions you can take that still move you forward. Remember how even small wins can trigger the brain's reward system? This isn't just about willpower. It's about working with your brain's natural wiring to make change feel safe and rewarding.

The beauty of micro-goals is that they strip away pressure and perfectionism, making it easy to follow through, especially on days when you feel tired or uninspired. They're so manageable that even on a chaotic morning or a stressful night, you can pull them off. To create your own micro-goals, start with something you want to improve, say, better hydration, more movement, or less stress. Now, shrink it down to the smallest action that would still count. The formula is simple: "After [trigger], I will [tiny action] for [time or reps]." For example, if your bigger goal is to meditate for twenty minutes, four times a week, you could start with, "After I sit at my desk, I will take three deep breaths." You might be surprised how much easier it is to commit to thirty seconds of stretching than to an hour-long yoga class. But as you gradually increase your mini-goals, you are getting closer to the bigger ones. Templates like this help you tailor actions to fit your lifestyle, not some ideal version of yourself who never gets busy or distracted.

Celebrating micro-wins is what keeps the momentum rolling. Every time you complete a small action, mark it down—a calendar checkmark, a sticker, or a quick note in your phone app. These visible reminders cue up your brain's reward system and reinforce the positive behavior. One reader shared how she started with just one minute of meditation each day. At first, it felt almost laughably simple, but as she saw her checkmarks pile up on the calendar, she began to feel proud of her effort. Within a month, she naturally expanded to five minutes, then ten. She didn't need to force herself because the growing streak made her want to keep going. That's the success spiral of each mini win fueling the next.

Momentum is addictive in the best way. The more you experience success, the more confident and motivated you become. This positive feedback loop is essential for adults juggling real-life demands because it creates an upward cycle instead of a pattern of frustration and quitting. You don't have to wait for some big breakthrough. Every checkmark is proof you're moving forward.

When energy runs high or time frees up unexpectedly, you can level up your micro-goal by stretching it a bit further. Maybe your two-minute walk turns into ten because you feel good and the weather's perfect. Or your daily gratitude list grows from one item to three. Let these expansions happen naturally—never as punishment for missing a bigger goal before, but as an expression of genuine enthusiasm.

If you want to see these strategies work in your own life, try mapping out three micro-goals for the week ahead using the formula: "After [trigger], I will [tiny action] for [time/minimum reps]." Track them with a visual cue like a calendar on the fridge or a tracking app on your phone. Watch how quickly those tiny wins add up and notice how your confidence grows with every checkmark.

THE HABIT RESET: TROUBLESHOOTING WHEN LIFE GETS MESSY

Real life has a way of wrecking even the best-laid plans. You might be on a roll with your new routine, then out of nowhere, the holiday season hits with its travel and endless gatherings, or work piles up to the ceiling. Sometimes, a family emergency pulls you away from your schedule. Maybe you catch a cold, or your kid wakes up sick in the middle of the night. These disruptions are not rare. They're part of being human. Over the years, we have seen so many people start strong, only to get thrown off course by a single unexpected event. There was one reader who wrote to us feeling so defeated after a week-long vacation. She'd set aside her habits for just a few days, but coming back felt like trying to climb a mountain in flip-flops. It's easy to think you've lost all your progress or that you never had the discipline in the first place. But the truth is, everyone faces setbacks. If you've struggled to keep habits going during chaos, you are absolutely not alone.

Getting back on track doesn't mean punishing yourself or overhauling everything overnight. Instead, a simple habit reset process can help. It starts with reflection, not self-critique. Ask yourself, "What got in the way?" Was it travel, extra stress, illness, or simply too much on your plate? Pinpointing the real disruptor helps you move forward without shame. Next, focus on just one micro-goal you can restart today. Not everything—just something small and doable. Maybe it's just doing a plank for thirty seconds or packing a healthy snack for work. The point is not to pick up where you left off at your peak, but to find the easiest re-entry point. Then, celebrate your first win back. Give yourself credit for simply showing up again. That first action is proof that you haven't given up; you're just recalibrating.

Habits can survive disruption when you allow them to adapt. Flexibility is key here. If a morning walk gets skipped because of rain or an early meeting, don't throw out the habit entirely. Instead, use an if/then plan: "If I miss my morning walk, then I'll do a three-minute cardio workout before my shower." This kind of backup plan gives you options, not excuses. Maybe it's swapping an outdoor run for a YouTube workout in your living room when the weather turns nasty. Or if your healthy lunches get derailed by last-minute deadlines, you shift to prepping something simple after dinner instead of at dawn. Habits aren't all or nothing, and they can flex with your day.

When life feels like it's spinning out of control, shrinking your habits is much better than scrapping them altogether. Rather than feeling defeated by missing a big workout or skipping meal prep for the week, ask what's the minimum action you can still take, no matter how small. This keeps the habit alive and makes it much easier to ramp up again when things settle down. Adaptation, because life gives you a little more than you can handle, does not mean failure. See it as a sign of your resilience and self-awareness.

Being gentle with yourself during these resets matters more than most people realize. Setbacks are normal. What actually predicts long-term change isn't never slipping up. It's how you respond when things go sideways. Studies show that those who are able to handle setbacks are 31 percent more productive when handling stressful situations and three times more inclined to maintain their sense of well-being (Applied Behavioral Holistic Health, n.d.). Instead of beating yourself up, try this script: "I'm proud of myself for coming back." Say it out loud if it helps, because returning after a break takes courage and determination.

We have talked to plenty of adults who believed one missed week spelled the end of their efforts. Yet the truth is, every return strengthens your habit muscle even more than getting it right every single day would. Resilience grows each time you reset and restart, even if your steps feel shaky at first.

If you need a quick step-by-step reset plan, here's what works:

- **Step 1:** Pause without judgment. Recognize that you aren't giving up but taking a moment to see what went wrong and reminding yourself that sometimes it's just part of life.
- **Step 2:** Name what happened. Either write down your thoughts or at least take a few minutes to decide exactly what happened. This is a chance to see the bigger picture and understand yourself better without blaming yourself.
- **Step 3:** Address your basic needs. Don't forget the foundations of your health. Perhaps you need to catch up on some sleep or handle your stress levels so that you aren't trying to pour from an empty cup.
- **Step 4:** Calm your nervous system. Do something that allows your body and mind to rest, such as a walk in nature or a warm bath.
- **Step 5:** Reframe your story. Turn the negative self-talk into something more realistic with the strategies we saw before, like letting go of perfectionism or adding yet to the end of your sentence.
- **Step 6:** Reconnect with your why. Go back to why you wanted to take control of your wellness to rediscover your motivation.
- **Step 7:** Set your mini-goal and commit to small actions.

As this chapter closes, remember that real habit-building isn't about perfection or streaks. It's about flexibility and kindness when things inevitably get messy. Your routines will change as life changes, and that's okay. The true win is learning how to reset and keep going, even after disruptions knock you sideways. In the next chapter, we'll dig into nutrition, the real-world way, so you can build eating habits that flex with your life.

4

NUTRITION REBUILT

Flexible, Real-World Eating and Meal Building for Any Schedule or Budget

How often do you stand in front of your fridge after a long day, tired and hungry, with no plan in sight? The takeout menu calls your name, but you want something that leaves you feeling good, not sluggish or guilty. This is where the Plate Blueprint steps in. Instead of memorizing complicated recipes or worrying about the perfect meal, you get a flexible, visual guide that takes the guesswork out of eating. Imagine a simple plate divided into three sections—one for protein, one for antioxidants, and one for carbs. That's it. No intricate math, no fancy gadgets, just an easy formula you can plug into any meal, anywhere.

MACROS MADE SIMPLE: PERSONALIZING NUTRITION WITHOUT OBSESSION

If you feel lost in all the talk about carbs, protein, and fat, collectively called macros, we know the feeling. Diet trends and social media often make macros seem complicated, but they're essentially the basics of what your food is made of. Carbohydrates are your body's quick energy source, found in pasta, rice, fruits, and potatoes. Protein builds and repairs muscle and is essential for many of the processes in the body, showing up in eggs, chicken, beans, fish, and yogurt. Despite outdated fears, fat is vital for brain health, hormones, and storing energy. You'll get it from nuts, seeds, avocado, cheese, and olive oil (Streit 2021). These three work together to fuel you, support daily functions, and help you feel satisfied.

When the body doesn't receive enough of these nutrients, especially in the form of protein-energy undernutrition, it begins to compensate by breaking down its own tissues to meet basic energy demands. Over time, this leads to muscle wasting, weakness, impaired immunity, and reduced organ function, as the body prioritizes survival over long-term health. On the other hand, when macronutrients are consumed in excess, particularly without corresponding physical activity, the body stores the surplus energy as fat in adipose tissue. Initially, this storage helps the body regulate energy availability. However, when storage capacity is exceeded, fat cells expand and contribute to chronic, low-grade inflammation. This metabolic imbalance is strongly linked to noncommunicable diseases (NCDs) such as type 2 diabetes, heart disease, and stroke (Cleveland Clinic 2022c). Maintaining a healthy balance of macronutrients, therefore, is not just about energy. It's about supporting overall metabolic health and preventing both deficiency and excess-related illnesses.

How you balance your macros is personal, so watch out for people who say you need X percentage of one and Y grams of another. If your day is physically active, like a teacher constantly on the move, you may need more carbohydrates. A runner training for a race will want extra carbs and protein to fuel practice and recovery. Parents chasing kids or multitasking may find that a bit of extra healthy fat (like avocado or nut butter) keeps their energy steady. There's no universal ideal macro split. Instead, pay attention to how you feel after meals. Are you satisfied or still hungry? Do you feel energized or crash later? If you're sluggish, try having more protein early or adding complex carbs.

Consider the experience of someone close to us who struggled with persistent morning fatigue, mistakenly believing it had no remedy. The root of the issue lay in her breakfast choices, which heavily leaned toward carbohydrates, consisting solely of toast and jam, without the balance of fats and proteins. The introduction of protein-rich Greek yogurt and almonds into her morning routine marked a big turn-around, enhancing her focus and sustaining her energy well into the afternoon.

Tweaking your macros isn't about tracking every bite or downloading a complicated app. Try easy upgrades: Toss chickpeas or grilled chicken on a salad for more protein, switch white rice for brown or quinoa, or add nuts to yogurt. These small changes help you feel fuller longer, without obsessing over every number or making drastic changes.

Above all, experiment to see what combinations help you feel good and satisfied. Notice shifts in your energy, mood, or hunger, and be curious. If lunch leaves you drained, add or swap a macro next time. No need for obsession, just stay observant and find what works for you.

SO, WHAT ABOUT MICRONUTRIENTS?

Micronutrients are vitamins and minerals that the body requires in small amounts but are vital for growth, development, immunity, and overall health. Unlike macronutrients, they don't provide energy, but they play key roles in metabolic processes, nerve function, bone health, and the production of enzymes and hormones. Some of the most essential micronutrients include vitamin D, vitamin B12, iron, calcium, iodine, and zinc. Because the body cannot produce micronutrients on its own (except for vitamin D), they must be obtained through a well-balanced diet (Jarai 2024).

Different foods are rich in different micronutrients. For example, vitamin D is found in fortified dairy products and egg yolks, and can also be synthesized through sunlight exposure. Vitamin B12, essential for red blood cell formation and nerve health, is mostly found in animal products like meat, fish, and dairy. Iron, crucial for oxygen transport in the blood, is present in red meat, lentils, and spinach. Calcium, needed for strong bones and teeth, is found in milk, cheese, and green leafy vegetables. Iodine, necessary for thyroid function, is often found in iodized salt and seafood. Zinc, which supports immunity and wound healing, is abundant in nuts, seeds, meat, and whole grains (Espinosa-Salas & Gonzalez-Arias 2023).

A deficiency in any of these micronutrients can lead to noticeable health problems. Low vitamin D can cause fatigue, bone pain, and weakened immunity. Iron deficiency often results in anemia, causing tiredness, pale skin, and shortness of breath. Vitamin B12 deficiency can lead to neurological symptoms like tingling in the hands and feet or memory issues. Calcium deficiency may contribute to brittle bones or muscle cramps. Iodine deficiency can cause goiter or slow metabolism, and zinc deficiency may lead to delayed healing, hair loss, or increased infections (Espinosa-Salas & Gonzalez-Arias 2023). Recognizing these signs early and correcting dietary intake—or supplementing when necessary—can prevent long-term health issues and restore balance.

THE ROLE OF ANTIOXIDANTS IN YOUR DIET

Antioxidants are powerful compounds that help protect the body from damage caused by free radicals, which are unstable molecules that are naturally produced during metabolism, exposure to pollution, UV rays, or toxins. When free radicals accumulate in the body, they can cause oxidative stress, damaging cells, proteins, and DNA. This damage is linked to aging and over fifty chronic diseases, including cancer, heart disease, and neurodegenerative conditions like Alzheimer's. Antioxidants work by neutralizing free radicals, essentially donating an electron to stabilize them and prevent further cellular harm (Tumilaar et al. 2024).

There are many types of antioxidants, both produced by the body and obtained through diet. Vitamin C, found in citrus fruits, berries, and bell peppers, is a water-soluble antioxidant that helps neutralize free radicals in the blood. Vitamin E, found in nuts, seeds, and leafy greens, is fat-soluble and protects cell membranes. Other key antioxidants include selenium (in Brazil nuts and seafood), beta-carotene (in carrots, sweet potatoes, and spinach), and polyphenols (plant compounds). You can take advantage of a little red wine and green tea for flavonoids (Better Health Channel 2024).

Herbs and spices are often overlooked but are among the richest sources of antioxidants. Turmeric contains curcumin, a compound with strong antioxidant and anti-inflammatory properties. Cinnamon, cloves, oregano, chili powder, parsley, and ginger are all loaded with natural compounds that fight oxidative stress (Todd 2021). Adding these herbs and spices to your meals not only enhances flavor but also boosts your body's ability to combat free radicals. Incorporating a colorful variety of plant-based foods and seasonings into your daily diet is one of the best strategies to maintain a strong antioxidant defense system and support overall health.

PERSONALIZING YOUR PLATE BLUEPRINT

The magic of the Plate Blueprint is its adaptability. No matter your morning rush or late-night craving, you can mix and match what's on hand. For breakfast, grab a bowl and toss in Greek yogurt (protein), some berries (antioxidants), and oats (carbs). If you're racing out the door, try a slice of whole grain bread with nut butter and a banana. Lunch doesn't have to be a sad desk salad. You could go with rotisserie chicken (protein), steamed broccoli (antioxidants), and a scoop of left-over rice (carbs). Even dinner can be simple: Sauté whatever veggies are left in your fridge, add canned beans, and wrap it all in a tortilla. The blueprint isn't about perfection. It's about building meals that fit what you actually have and like, and with the time you have available.

One of the best parts? This method works for any budget. You don't need to buy specialty items or shop at expensive stores. Frozen veggies stand in for fresh when money or time is tight. Canned beans, eggs, or tofu are more affordable protein sources. Brown rice, pasta, or potatoes fill out the carbs portion without draining your wallet. Swaps are always possible. Choose lentils for plant-based days, or gluten-free grains if needed. The Plate Blueprint allows you to personalize meals whether you're cooking solo, feeding picky kids, or sharing with roommates.

Let's talk about grocery shopping, because decision fatigue at the store is real. Instead of wandering the aisles hoping for inspiration, stick with a basic list of staples that fit into your plate model. Think eggs or tofu, mixed greens, apples, carrots, canned beans, whole grain wraps, and brown rice. These core ingredients can be stretched into dozens of combinations throughout the week. Batch-buying proteins and starches lets you freeze extras for quick defrosting later. Pre-chopped veggies, fresh or frozen, are total time-savers and reduce the temptation to order out just because you're tired. What's more, frozen veggies reduce the risk of food wastage, further helping the budget.

Eating out or grabbing food on the go doesn't have to derail your efforts either. When you're looking at a restaurant menu, scan for plates that hit all three sections: protein (grilled chicken, eggs, fish), antioxidants (side salad, steamed vegetables), and carbs (rice, pasta, potatoes). If portions are huge, split the meal or take half home for later. Cafeterias and convenience stores can work too. Look for hard-boiled eggs or cheese sticks (protein), a piece of fruit (antioxidants), and some whole grain crackers (carbs). Even gas stations offer yogurt cups and bananas these days.

Interactive: Build-Your-Own Plate Blueprint

Draw a circle on paper and divide it into three equal wedges. Label them Protein, Antioxidants, and Carbs. Under each section, list ten foods you actually enjoy that fit there. Mix favorites with what's affordable or available now. Keep this visual near your fridge or meal prep area as a cheat sheet when planning meals or shopping.

Instead of fussing over calories or perfect portions, use this visual as your anchor. You'll always know how to pull together something balanced, no matter how hectic life gets or how empty your pantry seems. The Plate Blueprint frees you from rigid meal plans by celebrating flexibility and making real-world eating work for real people.

MINDFUL EATING AND ENJOYING YOUR FOOD

Mindful eating means being fully present with your food, noticing what you eat and how your body feels before, during, and after meals. It's about engaging all your senses with each bite, smelling toast, feeling the crunch of an apple, or savoring the warmth of soup. This is about truly tasting your meals and tuning into your body's cues. Research has shown that when eating mindfully, you become more aware of hunger and fullness, helping prevent overeating and that uncomfortable stuffed feeling. The same research highlighted how mindful eating can reduce emotional eating (The Nutrition Source 2020). You may notice the emotions you bring to eating, such as stress, boredom, sadness, or celebration, so you don't use food as a mindless escape. Mindless snacking is common (think about eating chips without really tasting them), but mindful eating brings awareness. You savor the salt, the crunch, the satisfaction, and can stop eating when you're genuinely full, not just when the food is gone.

To practice mindful eating, slow down before a meal. Sit down instead of eating on the go. Take a few deep breaths and check in with your hunger: Are you eating because you're hungry, or simply because food is available? Before each bite, observe your food's color, aroma, and texture. Chew slowly, fully tasting each mouthful, and appreciate where your food comes from. If distractions like your phone or the TV pop up, gently bring your focus back to your meal (Willard 2022). Remind yourself: "I'm here with my meal, noticing each bite." At first, this may feel awkward, but with practice, it becomes a habit.

Food guilt is another challenge, a voice that labels pizza as bad or dessert as cheating. This all-or-nothing thinking actually causes more stress than the foods themselves. Instead of banning foods that trigger guilt or shame after eating them, practice self-compassion and give yourself permission. Swap "I shouldn't eat this" for "I'm allowed to enjoy this food. I'll savor it slowly." Allowing yourself to mindfully eat your favorite treat can reduce its power over you. For example, one reader stopped bingeing on cookies after giving herself permission to enjoy one mindfully whenever she wished. It turned out she needed less to feel satisfied, with no guilt attached.

Emotional or stress eating is normal. Everyone does it at some point. The goal isn't to force yourself to stop immediately but to bring awareness and kindness to the habit. When cravings hit, pause to consider your emotions: Are you tired, lonely, anxious? Jotting down your feelings can help. Ask yourself if food is truly what you need or if another comforting activity like journaling, listening to music, or calling a friend might feel better.

MEAL PREP HACKS FOR REAL LIFE: FROM SOLO LIVING TO BUSY FAMILIES

Meal prep sounds great in theory, but real life rarely looks like those perfect social media photos. Most of us feel too busy or tired to chop veggies for an hour on Sunday, let alone cook a week's worth of meals from scratch. The myth that you need to dedicate half your weekend to prepping food can actually stop you before you even start. Instead, meal prep can be something flexible and forgiving. Even twenty minutes on a Sunday can set you up for less chaos all week. For example, you might just wash fruit, portion out a few snacks, and cook a batch of rice or pasta. That's enough to take the edge off weekday meal stress and make healthier choices automatically.

Your lifestyle shapes what works best for prepping ahead. If you're cooking for yourself, simplicity is king. Think about your base plus a topping. Cook a pot of quinoa or brown rice, roast a tray of mixed veggies, and prepare a protein like chicken, tofu, or beans. Then combine them in different ways throughout the week: grain bowl on Monday, salad on Tuesday, wrap on Wednesday. Don't forget how different combinations of herbs and spices can change one staple greatly. For example, a chicken breast with lemon, ginger, and honey is completely different when you swap the additional ingredients for soya sauce and garlic. You may want to double recipes and use leftovers as lunch, or freeze the leftovers for when time is short. For families, sheet pan dinners are gold. You toss everything (chicken, potatoes, carrots, broccoli, as just one example) onto a tray, bake, and portion out meals for a few days. Freezer bag smoothie kits are another time-saver. Just dump fruit, greens, and seeds into bags so you can blend and go any morning.

Sustainability is all about finding shortcuts that match your reality. Automate what you can—set up a recurring grocery delivery, or at least use a saved list for staples to cut down on decision fatigue. Rotating meal themes takes planning off your plate. You could try themes like

Meatless Monday, Taco Tuesday, and Sheet Pan Saturday. Keep it playful and low-pressure. Cooking with kids or roommates can turn meal prep into bonding time instead of a chore. Give everyone a small job, even if it's just washing produce or setting up containers.

Of course, obstacles pop up. Maybe you just don't get to prepping this week, or the family rebels against last week's menu. When you miss your usual prep, do a quick reset. Scan your fridge and pantry for ready-to-use staples. Scramble eggs with spinach for dinner, microwave some frozen veggies with canned beans and salsa as a quick lunch, or throw together sandwiches and apples for the next day's lunch boxes. Boredom can sneak in, too. If you're tired of the same old meals, try one new sauce or seasoning blend to mix things up without starting from scratch. Don't let picky eaters derail your efforts. Offer build-your-own options by setting out the ingredients separately so everyone can assemble their own bowl or plate. If you fall off the wagon one week (or one month), don't sweat it. Simply start again with whatever feels manageable now. A small effort today saves you from food stress tomorrow.

As you wrap your head around these real-world hacks, remember that every bit of planning helps keep healthy eating within reach. Whether you're flying solo or feeding a crowd, meal prep can fit your life instead of taking it over. In the next chapter, we'll explore how movement can be just as flexible, because nutrition is only one part of building a strong foundation for wellness.

5

MOVEMENT THAT FITS

Exercise for Every Body and Schedule

Chances are you've experienced it: Hours at your desk, tight shoulders, heavy legs, and before you know it, most of the day has slipped by with barely any movement. Modern routines encourage prolonged sitting, which research connects with fatigue, aches, and major health risks like poor heart health, diabetes, depression, and even a shorter lifespan (Katella 2019). It may seem harmless, but sitting for long stretches actually signals your body to power down, slow metabolism, and ramp up inflammation.

DESKERCIZE AND DAILY MOVEMENT

And while regular workouts are good, long hours of sitting can still counteract those benefits. Our bodies need movement throughout the day, not just during planned exercise. According to physical therapist Olivia Rousseau, if you don't move every thirty minutes in your job, it's considered sedentary, and she recommends moving one or two minutes every thirty minutes (MU Health Care 2024). That's why movement snacks, brief, frequent activity breaks, are gaining popularity. Instead of saving all movement for gym sessions, you weave thirty seconds to five minutes of activity bursts into your daily routine. Research shows that movement snacks can be more beneficial than one hour at the gym (Nourkhalaj 2024).

Take a typical morning full of video calls. You may not be able to go out for a run, but you can fit in some quick "deskercize" moves at your workspace and with no special gear required. Try a five-minute chair stretch: Sit tall with feet flat, reach both arms overhead, fingers interlaced, and stretch upward, holding for a deep breath. Next, lean to each side with one arm overhead for a side stretch. Roll your shoulders backward in large circles, five or six times each way. Then, cross your right ankle over your left knee, lean forward for a hip stretch, and switch legs. Finish with a gentle twist: Sitting upright, hold the back of the chair with your right hand and your right thigh with your left hand, gently twisting to look over your shoulder, switching after a breath. This routine is quicker than checking social media and can instantly revive your body.

Try standing calf raises while waiting for coffee or lunch. Hold on to your desk for balance, rise onto your toes, and lower down slowly. Repeat ten times to wake up tired legs. For posture and focus, add seated spinal rotations: Sit tall, cross arms on your chest, and gently twist side to side. This can help counteract slouching and lift your energy.

Incorporate movement into daily tasks to make staying active easy. Walk during phone calls with headphones, or, if that's not an option, stand and shift your weight instead of sitting still. At night during TV commercials, use the time to do squats, lunges, or march in place. Even chores count, and you can make them more enjoyable. Put on music while folding laundry and sneak in a dance or calf raise between loads.

Consistency is easier with reminders. Set an hourly timer or use a smartwatch to prompt you to stand, stretch, or walk for two minutes. Apps like Break Time, Move, or Stand Up! can nudge you to take stretch breaks (Family Living 2025). Prefer analog? Use a printed habit tracker on your desk to check off each movement break and watch your progress grow for motivation.

Accountability helps, too. Text a friend or colleague when you take movement breaks and encourage each other. If you share a workspace, suggest a daily stretch o'clock for everyone to take a quick group break. No judgment, just movement and maybe some laughs.

Interactive: Build Your Personal Deskercize Routine

Grab your notes app or journal and jot down three times you typically feel sluggish (after lunch, before late meetings, or post-bedtime routine). Next to each, pick a movement snack such as thirty seconds of jumping jacks, jogging on the spot, or a five-minute Zumba session. Place these reminders on your monitor or set calendar alerts as prompts. At the end of the day, check off each break completed with a focus on improvement, not perfection.

CUSTOMIZABLE WORKOUTS: QUICK WINS FOR HOME, OFFICE, OR TRAVEL

Movement doesn't need to be complicated, expensive, or tied to a gym. Life throws enough curveballs with work deadlines, travel, unpredictable weather, kids, or just a tiny living space, and traditional workout plans rarely survive all that. What you need is flexibility. You need a way to build your own workouts that fit right into your real world, not someone else's perfect setup. We want you to feel in control, whether you've got ten spare minutes or only a patch of carpet between your sofa and coffee table.

Building a workout that works for you starts with the pick-one-from-each-column blueprint. Take your journal and draw a chart with four columns: Upper body, lower body, core, and cardio. Below, you can find examples of excellent exercises for each with videos.

- **Upper Body:** Back rows, bicep curls, chest press, tricep extension, shoulder press, and cross-body front raise.
  - https://www.youtube.com/watch?v=xxVRCzT2a1E
- **Lower Body:** Squats, sumo squats, deadlifts, calf raises, reverse lunges, and glute bridges.
  - https://www.youtube.com/watch?v=zZ8tWnE8kzQ

- **Core:** Tabletop crunches, leg drop motion, plank, plank hip dip, Russian twists, straight leg dead bugs, and oblique crunches.
  - https://www.youtube.com/watch?v=Cnmy08JgakM
- **Cardio:** Hand to floor squat jumps, single knee drive jump, three-point lunge, lunge jumps, sprawl, and reverse crunch.
  - https://www.youtube.com/watch?v=kZDvg92tTMc

Once you've picked a move or two from each group, put them together for a circuit. This could be as simple as thirty seconds per movement with a short breather in between, or you could count reps if you prefer structure, say 10–15 reps of each. The beauty of tailoring your workouts like this is that they fit into your timeframes perfectly. For the days you are pressed for time, you can choose fewer reps. If you find yourself blessed with a little extra time, you can add an additional exercise or increase the time. What's more, with plenty of variety to choose from, your workouts won't become boring.

Equipment, or lack of it, should never be a barrier. A towel can double as a slider on tile or wood floors for hamstring curls or mountain climbers. Resistance bands travel light and work almost anywhere. They're perfect for rows or biceps curls when dumbbells aren't handy. Speaking of dumbbells, water bottles make an ideal replacement. If you're on the road and stuck in a hotel room, use the edge of the bed for triceps dips or split squats. In a tiny apartment? Chair squats, wall sits, and standing calf raises all fit within arm's reach. The backpack trick is one of our favorites. Load it up with whatever's heavy but safe (books, laundry detergent) and hug it while doing squats, presses, or rows.

For those days when motivation is scraping the bottom of the barrel, or when you're just so slammed that even thinking about exercise feels like too much, micro-goals keep you moving. We call these win workouts because they count no matter how short. Choose three moves, maybe squats, push-ups (against the wall if needed), and a plank hold for fifteen seconds. Set a timer for five minutes and see how many rounds you can complete without rushing. Or put on your favorite upbeat song and move however you like, dance in your socks, shadowbox in the kitchen, or sway while folding laundry. One study showed how 98 percent of the 1,000 participants experienced improved mood, confidence, and compassion, as well as letting go of distressing thoughts when practicing free-form dancing (UCLA Health 2021).

Travel often leaves us stiff and drained, so a five-minute yoga flow for recovery is recommended. You could try cat-cow stretches for your back, neck, and shoulders, downward dog to stretch your legs and back, or child's pose to breathe out the stress. If you're feeling ambitious, toss in some gentle lunges or standing side bends. These short sessions break up long flights or car rides and help you feel like yourself again. Don't forget there are plenty of free apps that have a range of exercises, especially for quick workouts, like Nike Training Club where you can select types of workouts, areas of the body, intensity, and duration (Nike Training Club, n.d.). Another option many of us use is FitOn. Aside from workouts, there are also meditation sessions and help with weekly goals (FitOn, n.d.). Having these options on your phone is particularly handy when you are traveling.

Listening to your body is more important than any plan. There's no prize for pushing through pain or ignoring fatigue. On days your energy is low or old injuries flare up, swap high-impact moves for gentler options. Step touches replace jumping jacks without stressing your joints. Chair squats offer support if balance feels shaky. Wall push-ups are friendly on wrists and shoulders, but still strengthen your chest and arms. If something doesn't feel right, please stop. There's power in adjusting instead of forcing yourself through discomfort.

Some days will demand more adaptation than others, especially if you're managing chronic pain or recovering from illness. Give yourself permission to take it slow and modify further. Seated marches from your couch count as movement, so does rolling your shoulders or stretching gently at your desk. Set a goal for consistency and self-respect.

With these blueprints and tweaks, you create movement that fits into whatever life hands you, whether that's busy mornings, work trips, small spaces, low motivation days, or even achy joints. It's about making exercise accessible so you never feel shut out by a lack of equipment, space, time, or energy. You hold the power to adapt every workout to your needs, not the other way around, and every effort is worth celebrating.

OVERCOMING EXERCISE PLATEAUS AND BOREDOM: MAKING MOVEMENT JOYFUL

Everyone hits the wall at some point, where your workouts just stop delivering the same results. Maybe you used to feel stronger or more energized, but suddenly, progress stalls, or you even start to dread exercise. This is what's called a plateau, and, despite being frustrating, it's not a sign of failure but a normal part of the body's adaptation process. Your muscles and nervous system get used to the same old moves, and over time, they stop responding with the same gains in strength or stamina (Cronkleton 2022). If you're bored or frustrated, it's not your fault.

Variety is your secret weapon. If you usually do high-intensity interval training (HIIT), try switching to a slower-paced workout like Pilates or a steady bike ride for a week or two. Mixing up movement styles can wake up sleepy muscles and refresh your brain. You might find that taking a challenge week once every month or two, where you add totally new exercises, snaps you out of a rut and brings back that feeling of accomplishment. Even shifting the order of your usual moves, trying new environments, or simply resting for a few days can spark new growth. You can also try progressive overload to increase the duration, reps, or intensity of your workouts.

But breaking through plateaus isn't just about mixing up routines. It's about finding joy again in movement. So many adults grew up with exercise as punishment. Run laps for messing up in gym class, or count calories to earn dessert. That mindset sticks and makes working out feel like a chore instead of self-care. The trick is to focus on what genuinely brings you pleasure. Not everyone enjoys running or lifting weights, and that's okay. Dance workouts in your living room can lift your mood instantly, even if you have two left feet. Hiking allows you to connect with nature while moving at your own speed. Recreational sports, think tennis, ultimate frisbee, even dodgeball, make movement social and playful, not just sweaty and serious. Pick one new activity each month to try, whether it's roller skating, swimming laps, or learning a round of golf. Switch the focus to rediscovering what makes you smile.

Movement doesn't have to look like traditional exercise at all. The concept of movement as play is powerful, especially for those who've lost touch with fun physical activity. Remember childhood games like hopscotch, tag, and climbing trees? Adults need to play just as much as kids do. It's a secret ingredient for motivation and stress relief as you stay in the present moment (Trainer O&O Coach 2021). Social fitness takes this even further: When you move with others, you get accountability plus laughter and connection. Organize a virtual group workout with friends who live far away—Zoom yoga sessions or online dance parties are surprisingly energizing. Local walking or cycling groups can introduce you to new people and make sticking with movement much easier. If you have family at home, invite them for after-dinner walks or create backyard obstacle courses. Turning exercise into a group event transforms "I should" into "I want to."

Real stories always carry more weight than generic advice, so let me share a few from readers who changed their relationship with movement for good. One person wrote in about crippling gym anxiety. She hated feeling watched and judged, so she gave up on working out entirely for years. Then, after discovering online dance workouts she could do in her bedroom with nobody watching, she started moving just for the joy of it. She now looks forward to those sessions, never worrying about how she looks, only how she feels. Another reader suffered an injury that made high-impact activities impossible. Instead of quitting altogether, he experimented with gentle yoga and realized he could still get stronger and more flexible without pain. That sense of accomplishment rebuilt his confidence and made him excited to keep moving.

For many adults, redefining exercise as self-care instead of punishment is a game-changer. It takes practice to let go of old beliefs about what counts as real fitness or what your body should be able to do. Progress looks different for everyone. Sometimes it's running farther than last week, other times it's simply showing up for yourself after a tough day.

If you're feeling stuck, ask yourself: What activity have I always wanted to try but never did? What type of movement actually makes me laugh or forget about time? Who do I enjoy spending time with who might move with me? Experiment until you land on something that genuinely excites you, even if it changes every season.

As we conclude this chapter, we see that variety and playfulness turn movement into something you look forward to instead of another obligation on your list. When exercise becomes joyful again, sticking with it gets easier, and your body and mind will thank you.

Looking ahead, movement is only one pillar of wellness. Next up, we'll dive into sleep, the underrated superpower that fuels every effort you make toward better health.

6

SLEEP AS A SUPERPOWER

Restoring Energy in a 24/7 World

You know those nights when your head hits the pillow and your brain suddenly wants to replay every awkward moment you've ever had? Or worse, it starts composing tomorrow's to-do list in vivid, anxious detail. If you feel like sleep is something you're always chasing but never quite catching, you're in good company. In a world that worships productivity and celebrates the grind, restful sleep often gets shoved to the back burner until exhaustion catches up and refuses to be ignored. Sleep gives the brain a chance to repair. It's when our long-term memories are formed, and it's vital for the circulatory system, metabolism, the respiratory system, and the immune system (National Heart, Lung, and Blood Institute 2022). It makes little sense to work on your diet and activity levels only to abandon sleep!

SLEEP HYGIENE DEMYSTIFIED: BUILDING YOUR IDEAL WIND-DOWN RITUAL

Sleep hygiene is simply the set of habits and routines that prepare your brain and body to rest. This isn't just about being cozy, as there's real science behind it. Your brain relies on strong cues from your environment and your behaviors to start winding down. Your body relies on two key systems to manage when you feel awake and when you feel tired: sleep-wake homeostasis and your circadian rhythm. Sleep-wake homeostasis tracks the amount of time you've been awake—the longer you stay up, the stronger the internal drive to sleep becomes. If this system worked by itself, you'd feel most refreshed upon waking and steadily more tired as the day went on, naturally leading to sleep at night.

However, your circadian rhythm adds another layer to this regulation. This biological clock influences fluctuations in alertness and drowsiness over a twenty-four-hour period. Most adults, for instance, tend to experience noticeable dips in energy between 2 a.m. and 4 a.m., and again from 1 p.m. to 3 p.m., even if they've had plenty of rest (Johns Hopkins Medicine, n.d.). Maintaining a consistent sleep schedule can help reduce the impact of these daily energy slumps.

The timing of your circadian rhythm is controlled by a tiny cluster of cells in the brain known as the suprachiasmatic nucleus (SCN), found in the hypothalamus. This area responds to light signals picked up by your eyes. In the morning, exposure to light prompts the SCN to signal the release of cortisol and other hormones that promote wakefulness. As darkness falls, the SCN activates the pineal gland, which then produces melatonin, the hormone that helps you feel relaxed and ready for sleep. Together, these systems help maintain a stable and healthy sleep-wake cycle (Johns Hopkins Medicine, n.d.).

So what does a good wind-down look like? There's no universal prescription. The key is picking activities that help you shift from go mode to slow mode. For some, that might be reading a physical book, a real one, with pages you can turn, not another glowing screen that tricks your brain into thinking it's still daytime. Blue light from our devices prevents the production of melatonin, so all screens should be avoided. Others love gentle stretching or restorative yoga, which helps release tension from the day while signaling to muscles and joints that rest is near. Maybe you prefer listening to calming music or white noise. Certain sounds—rainfall, ocean waves, soft instrumental tracks—can lower your heart rate and create a soothing atmosphere. Aromatherapy is another favorite; just a little lavender or chamomile in a diffuser or pillow spray can nudge your senses toward relaxation. The idea isn't to do everything but to pick two or three calming rituals you genuinely enjoy and can repeat most nights. Ideally, your wind-down should last around thirty minutes (Suni 2024).

Environmental factors can sabotage even the best bedtime intentions. Light is a major culprit. Think about how streetlights or screens can keep your brain wired. Blackout curtains or even a comfortable eye mask can help block out unwanted brightness. Sound matters too. If you share your space with snorers, city noise, or unpredictable pets, try using a white noise machine or an app that masks disruptive sounds. Temperature also makes a huge difference. You may sleep best in a cool room with breathable bedding. If you wake up sweaty or shivering, tweak your blankets or pajamas until you find that sweet spot. Decluttering your sleep space can work wonders. It's hard to relax in a bedroom overflowing with laundry piles. Even if your home is tiny or shared with others, make your bed a calm zone by clearing nightstands and keeping clutter at bay.

Sometimes the biggest obstacles aren't physical but mental. You plan to get to bed early, but end up answering just one more email or scrolling social media into the wee hours. Maybe anxious thoughts refuse to quiet down once things get still. If you catch yourself feeling wired at bedtime, have a backup plan. Try a five-minute guided meditation (there are plenty of free options online) to help transition from anxiety to calm. If your mind keeps racing with worries or unfinished business, grab a journal and spend ten minutes offloading every nagging thought onto paper. It could be as simple as writing a to-do list for the next day. One study showed how those who wrote a to-do list fell asleep faster than those who wrote a list of completed activities. There is a technique called a brain dump that can reduce mental clutter. Set a timer for five minutes and spend that time literally dumping everything that's on your mind onto the paper (Somanathan 2025).

If/then plans may support moments of resistance. For example: "If I notice myself reaching for my phone after lights out, then I'll turn on a calming playlist instead." Or, "If I feel like I can't stop thinking about work, then I'll write down three things I did well today before closing my notebook." These small swaps retrain your habits without relying on sheer willpower.

Interactive: Build Your Custom Wind-Down Ritual

Take five minutes tonight and jot down two activities that help you relax (reading, stretching, music, aromatherapy, whatever feels right). Next, write one backup plan for nights when worry or restlessness shows up ("If my mind is busy, then I'll journal for ten minutes"). Stick this cheat sheet by your bed as a gentle reminder. Tweak as needed until your ritual feels like a true invitation for deep rest. Don't forget to use this reminder along with your wind-down. Each small step signals to your brain and body that it's safe to let go of the day and recharge for whatever tomorrow brings.

ADAPTING SLEEP SOLUTIONS: IRREGULAR SCHEDULES, SHIFT WORK, AND PARENTING

If you've ever tried to sleep while the sun blazes through the window or after your toddler woke you up three times before dawn, you know that "just get eight hours" advice doesn't cut it. Life runs on unpredictable rhythms for so many adults. There are shift workers, new moms and dads, caregivers, and anyone whose calendar isn't really their own. It's not just about feeling tired. There's frustration, a sense of falling behind, sometimes even guilt. You scroll articles online, see well-meaning advice that assumes a nine-to-five life, and wonder if anyone understands what your nights are really like.

We remember a night-shift nurse who shared her story with us. Her hospital schedule changed every week, and she'd swing between day and night shifts with barely a pause. She would come home when the world was waking up, exhausted but unable to wind down. Her room was bright, the neighbors were loud, and her body wanted breakfast when she needed sleep. She felt jealous of friends with regular routines and sometimes blamed herself for her constant fatigue. The truth is, our biology is wired for the sun. When your work or family needs flip that on its head, sleep becomes a puzzle that deserves real solutions, not shame.

For anyone working nights or inconsistent shifts, rest is all about controlling what you can. First, begin with the basics that we have already seen, particularly light and noise. If you live with others, try using a "sleep in progress" sign or negotiate quiet hours if possible. Caffeine is another tricky one. Sometimes it feels like the only thing keeping you alert at work, but it can stick around in your system for hours. Try to cut off coffee or energy drinks at least four hours before your planned rest time. You might crave that last cup at the end of a shift, but skipping it can make falling asleep easier. One trick many shift workers swear by is the sleep anchor. Pick one block of time in every twenty-four hours and try to keep it consistent, even if your schedule changes wildly. For example, maybe you always nap from 2 to 6 p.m., no matter what shift you're on. This gives your body at least one predictable window to settle into deeper rest and help your circadian rhythm (Glenn 2020).

Parenting and caregiving bring their own set of sleep challenges, ones that rarely get credit for how tough they are. Babies wake up crying, toddlers crawl into bed at 2 a.m., teens come home late, and sometimes your only quiet moment is after everyone else is asleep. Fragmented rest becomes the norm. If you have a partner, see if you can tag-team with alternate nights on duty or split the night into shifts so each of you gets at least one longer stretch of sleep now and then. Even single parents or solo caregivers can use creative swaps like trading sleep-ins with a friend or relative when possible or napping during kids' screen time. Please don't feel guilty for this. As parents, we know that when little people fall asleep, we look around at all the things that need to be done, but they will still be there later, and you will be a better parent if you are rested. Power naps work wonders if you keep them short and sweet, no more than twenty minutes (Gerrestsen 2024). This can help you avoid grogginess and still refresh your brain.

The guilt that creeps in when full nights are impossible can be heavy. It's easy to compare yourself to others or to some ideal version of adulthood where everyone sleeps eight hours in peace. Wellness isn't about hitting some mythical number every night. It's about making the best of what you've got. Every extra minute of rest is a win. The other day, we were talking about a reader who used to beat herself up after weeks of broken sleep with her newborn. She'd stare at the clock in frustration, feeling defeated when she couldn't piece together more than four hours at a time. Eventually, she stopped measuring herself against other parents whose babies were apparently already sleeping through the night and started celebrating small victories like a longer nap here, an early bedtime there, a rare morning when everyone slept in. That shift from "I failed again" to "Any progress counts" changed her entire mood and made her more patient with herself and her family.

There's no badge for suffering through exhaustion just to meet someone else's definition of healthy sleep. Some nights will be rough, while others will surprise you with unexpected ease. Allow yourself grace on both kinds of nights, and remember, a few extra minutes of rest can lead to less morning fog and a better mood by lunchtime. Your wellness builds over time from all the little adjustments and moments of self-compassion.

TRACKING PROGRESS BEYOND THE PILLOW: ENERGY, MOOD, AND RECOVERY

Some mornings you wake up with a clear head and a spark of energy, ready to take on the day. Other times, you drag yourself out of bed, groggy and irritable, feeling like sleep was just a rumor. It's easy to focus on how many hours you spent in bed and call it a night's work, but that number on the clock rarely tells the whole story. What truly matters is how rested you feel and how your sleep shapes your day, your energy, your mood, your ability to think clearly, and even your appetite. This is where tracking your sleep gets interesting, not just for the sake of data, but for finding patterns that actually matter to your life.

While you can use fancy gadgets or endless notifications from sleep apps, there's a simple, human way to check in. Pay attention to how you feel when you wake up. Try jotting down a quick morning check in a notebook or on your phone, something as basic as "How do I feel today?" or "What's my energy like right now?" You might use a 1–10 scale, with 1 being "please don't talk to me" and 10 being "unstoppable." Or, use words that make sense to you: sluggish, meh, sharp, restless, steady. These self-checks take less than a minute, and over time, these tiny notes give you a map of how you sleep.

Patterns start to emerge when you connect the dots across several days or weeks. Maybe you notice that every time you stay up scrolling through your phone, the next morning feels like walking through fog. Perhaps eating late or having an extra glass of wine means you're more irritable or distracted the next day. Some people spot that when they get even half an hour more rest, their workouts feel stronger or their patience stretches just a little further. Consider keeping a weekly energy/mood log where you rate your morning and evening energy, jot down how focused you felt at work or during chores, and mark any standout moods—good or bad.

Sleep isn't always predictable, though. You'll inevitably run into nights where rest just doesn't happen—stressful deadlines, restless kids, noisy neighbors, or simply tossing and turning for no clear reason. When that happens, instead of beating yourself up or trying to power through on caffeine alone, focus on gentle recovery strategies that help offset the sleep debt, the difference between the amount of sleep you get and the amount of sleep your body needs. For adults, this can be between seven and nine hours (Covenant Health 2024). Start with movement. Even a slow ten-minute walk outside can help shake off grogginess and signal to your body that it's time to reset. Natural light, especially sun exposure in the morning, helps recalibrate your body clock and can boost alertness (Suni 2024). Hydration matters too; after poor sleep, drink water before reaching for more coffee. Dehydration amplifies fatigue and makes it harder for your brain to function (Vasquez 2023).

Reflection makes progress stick. Once a month, pause and ask yourself, "What sleep change made the biggest difference this month?" It could be something as small as turning off screens earlier or saying no to late-night caffeine. Write it down somewhere, and consider what you want to keep or tweak going forward. These moments of honest review turn vague intentions into real habits.

Sleep isn't just about logging hours; it's about restoring what life takes out of us so we can show up as our best selves, even when things aren't perfect. Tracking how you feel, noticing patterns, bouncing back from rough nights, and building on small wins will transform bedtime from an afterthought into one of your strongest wellness tools. Appreciate how the last three chapters are intricately linked. A better diet can provide you with more energy, and with more energy, you will find exercising easier, and when you are more physically active, getting a good night's sleep becomes more likely!

As we close this chapter on sleep and its ripple effects across daily life, remember, meaningful change starts with noticing how rest feels in your body, how it shapes your day, and how small choices compound over time. Up next, we explore how managing stress transforms not only your nights but also every waking hour, unlocking resilience right where you need it most.

7

STRESS MASTERY

From Overwhelm to Resilience

You know that feeling when your phone won't stop pinging, inboxes pile up, and your shoulders tighten? Stress can hit fast, leaving you tense and frazzled. Powering through only makes things worse. Your body reacts with clenched jaws, a racing heart, and a restless mind. In these moments, you don't need a lengthy lecture or a spa, but quick, proven tools you can use wherever you are, at your desk, in your car, even in the bathroom at work.

UNDERSTANDING THE STRESS RESPONSE

We are going to go back to a little science before covering the strategies. We are living in a world that seems to accept stress as something normal. But with this mentality, we don't fully appreciate the damage high levels of stress can do to the body. Our intention with this section isn't to scare you. It's to make you realize that stress can't be ignored.

When the body perceives a threat, whether physical or emotional, it activates a well-coordinated stress response system designed to help us react quickly. This response begins in the limbic system, a set of brain structures that includes the amygdala, hippocampus, and hypothalamus, all of which are involved in processing emotions and memory. The amygdala, in particular, plays a critical role in detecting danger and signaling the hypothalamus to initiate the stress response (Cleveland Clinic 2024a).

The hypothalamus, acting as the command center, communicates with the autonomic nervous system (ANS) to trigger the "fight-or-flight" response. The ANS has two main branches: the sympathetic nervous system (SNS) and the parasympathetic nervous system (PNS). During stress, the SNS is activated, releasing adrenaline (epinephrine) and noradrenaline into the bloodstream. This leads to physiological changes such as increased heart rate, rapid breathing, dilated pupils, and a surge of glucose into the bloodstream for immediate energy (Harvard Health Publishing 2024).

If the stressor persists, the hypothalamus activates the HPA axis (hypothalamic-pituitary-adrenal axis), leading to the release of cortisol, the body's primary stress hormone. Cortisol helps sustain energy by regulating metabolism, immune function, and blood pressure. However, prolonged activation of this system, known as chronic stress, can dysregulate the limbic system, impair memory, increase anxiety, and suppress immune function. In fact, chronic stress is linked to the six leading causes of death in the US: heart disease, cancer, lung and respiratory disorders, accidental injuries, cirrhosis of the liver, and suicide (Pugle 2022).

The PNS later steps in to calm the body down, restoring homeostasis. This "rest-and-digest" state helps slow the heart rate and supports recovery after the perceived threat has passed, but this can take anywhere from twenty to sixty minutes to occur (Cherry 2024a). It might sound all doom and gloom, but there is one nerve in the body that can reduce stress in an instant. That nerve is going to be a key part of your quick strategies for dealing with stress.

THE RESILIENCE TOOLKIT: QUICK STRATEGIES FOR HIGH-PRESSURE MOMENTS

The vagus nerve is the tenth cranial nerve and the longest in the body. This nerve contains 75 percent of the parasympathetic nerve fibers. It passes your neck and then branches into the heart, lungs, abdomen, and digestive tract. It plays an essential role in your mood, heart rate, breathing, and digestion, to name a few (Cleveland Clinic 2022a). By stimulating your vagus nerve, you can activate the PNS to help the body calm down. Because the vagus nerve passes through the neck, and therefore the voice box, things like singing, humming, and gargling with water can naturally stimulate your vagus nerve. Cold exposure is another quick strategy. You could try holding a cold pack on your neck, submerging your face in cold water, or taking a plunge into a cold shower.

Finally, deep breathing can also stimulate the vagus nerve (Laderer 2024).

One of the fastest stress-busters is box breathing. Sit comfortably, hands in your lap. Inhale through your nose for four counts. Hold for four. Exhale through your mouth for four. Hold for another four. Picture tracing a box in your mind with each step—up as you inhale, across as you hold, down as you exhale, and across again as you pause. Repeat three to five times. Most people feel their heart rate slow and their mind quiet. Box breathing works anywhere, takes about a minute, and is barely noticeable (Migala 2024).

If stress hits as physical tension, such as hunched shoulders and a stiff neck, a quick body scan can reset you. Close your eyes (or lower your gaze if you prefer). Breathe deeply and focus on the top of your head. Notice any tension. Move your attention slowly down your forehead, jaw, shoulders, arms, chest, belly, hips, legs, and feet. At each spot, notice tightness and, if you find any, breathe into it and let it go a bit more with every breath. Three minutes is enough to soften clenched muscles and bring relief (Corliss, n.d.). You don't need silence or music, just a willingness to check in with yourself.

Build an emergency resilience kit with items and reminders that ground you. It might include a stress ball, calming scents (like lavender oil), headphones for favorite music, or a handwritten affirmation such as "This too shall pass." Keep your kit handy, whether that's in your bag, desk, or car's glove box.

Build-Your-Own Resilience Kit: Checklist

- Stress ball or handheld fidget
- Scented lotion or essential oil (lavender, citrus, peppermint)
- Affirmation card ("I am safe," "I've got this," "Breathe")
- Earbuds/headphones and a favorite calming playlist
- Small notebook or sticky notes for jotting down worries
- Cold pack or travel-sized facial spray
- Photo of someone or somewhere comforting

Physical cues show up before you consciously realize you're stressed. This can include clenched jaws, hunched shoulders, teeth grinding, and shallow breaths. Racing thoughts and irritability are also common signals. These are your body's early warnings. When you catch yourself sighing or rubbing your neck, pause and ask, "What am I feeling physically right now? Is there tension I can release?" The sooner you notice, the easier it is to diffuse stress before it explodes.

True recovery doesn't require a long break. Micro-recovery fits even the busiest day. After a tough conversation, stand up, stretch, or drink water before starting your next task. These mini-reset rituals help return your system from high alert to steady ground. Stress mastery isn't about overhauling your life, but using fast, routine-friendly tools to help you bounce back instead of burn out. Keep track of the effects each strategy has, perhaps with a 1 to 5 scale. Your stress-busting strategies have to be personal. Imagine if the smell of lavender stirs up bad memories? Trying lavender essential oils is just going to stress you out more. Once you have narrowed down the most effective strategies, you know you have your personalized toolkit.

MINDFUL MINUTES: INTEGRATING SHORT, EFFECTIVE PRACTICES INTO YOUR DAY

Mindfulness really gets a bad rap for being too "out there" or hippy, like you need a meditation cushion, incense, or a silent mountain retreat just to get started. In reality, mindfulness is simply the act of remaining in the present without feeling overwhelmed (Mindful 2025). If you think about it, all your stress and problems come from thinking about the past or worrying about the future. The present moment is a peaceful one. You don't have to set aside thirty minutes or even ten. Mindfulness can be squeezed into the smallest cracks of your day. You could be stopped at a red light, waiting in the checkout line, or brushing your teeth before bed. Those tiny, intentional pauses to engage your senses and keep you grounded can work wonders.

So, how can you be more mindful when you're sandwiched between work emails, errands, and a house full of responsibilities? Try this the next time you're waiting to pick up the kids or for your coffee to brew: Stop whatever else you're doing, let your hands rest in your lap, and breathe in deeply through your nose. Let your shoulders drop a notch. Now, notice what sounds you hear? How do your feet feel against the ground? Is your jaw tight? Can you relax it just a touch? On the next exhale, let go of any urge to rush. If your brain wanders (it will), gently bring it back to one thing you can sense right now.

Everyday routines hold hidden space for mindful moments, too. When washing your hands, instead of zoning out or making to-do lists in your mind, pay attention to the sensation of water on your skin. Notice the temperature, the feel and smell of the soap, and the sound of water splashing in the sink. Breathe slowly, letting the act become an anchor that pulls you out of autopilot for a few seconds. Teeth-brushing works just as well. Feel the bristles moving across your gums, taste the minty foam, hear the hum of the brush. If your mind skips ahead to tomorrow's schedule or yesterday's argument, don't judge or criticize yourself. Just bring it back to the present and finish up.

When stress builds or overwhelm creeps in, the 5-4-3-2-1 grounding technique can steady you fast. Pause wherever you are and mentally scan: What are five things I see? Four things I can touch? Three sounds I notice? Two smells in the air? One thing I can taste (even if it's only a hint of coffee on your tongue)? This quick inventory pulls you straight into your body and away from spiraling thoughts and counteracts the "fight-or-flight" response (Calm 2024). You don't have to do all five steps every time; just focusing on a few senses is enough to pull you out of your head and onto solid ground.

These mindful minutes really add up over time. Imagine each practice as a drip into an inner well of calm and resilience. At first, it might not seem like much, a few deep breaths here, a quick check-in there, but those moments begin to stack up. They form a buffer between you and daily chaos. There's a reader who shared how he started taking three mindful sips of coffee every morning before checking his phone or emails. At first, it felt awkward and even pointless. But after a month, he noticed those moments set the tone for his whole morning. He felt more present, less reactive, and surprisingly less rushed, even on busy days.

If you've ever felt too busy or skeptical about mindfulness, know that these short pauses aren't about changing who you are. They're about meeting yourself where you are, over and over again. Each mindful minute is a seed planted for more calm and resilience down the road, no cushion required. Give yourself credit for every pause, no matter how brief or imperfect it feels.

EMOTIONAL EATING AND STRESS AND TOOLS FOR BREAKING THE CYCLE

Stress intricately intertwines with our eating habits, extending far beyond mere willpower. Under tension, our bodies release cortisol, a stress hormone, triggering food cravings (Harvard Health Publishing 2012). Unfortunately, we rarely crave a nice piece of fruit in these moments. Instead, we reach for high-salt or sugary treats like chips, fries, or extra slices of cake. This response is not merely psychological but a physiological mechanism rooted in survival, a vestige from our ancestors who needed quick energy boosts to evade predators. In the modern context, these predators are replaced by office deadlines, challenging conversations, and overwhelming schedules. Consequently, after a stressful day, one might find oneself reaching for comfort food in the pantry, seeking not nourishment but solace and a semblance of control. This act of eating momentarily activates the brain's reward centers, providing immediate relief but soon followed by a crash, often accompanied by feelings of guilt or frustration.

To break out of autopilot eating, you need to spot your own patterns. Start by paying attention to when and where stress eating tends to hit hardest. Is it always late at night when the house finally goes quiet? Does it creep up after tense work calls or when you feel bored and restless at home? Maybe celebrations or even good news can kick off the urge to treat yourself. Tracking your triggers helps you see them coming before you're elbow-deep in a snack bag. Jot down the time, place, emotion, and food choice whenever you catch yourself reaching for comfort food. Over a week or two, look for patterns, like when maybe fatigue and late afternoon show up again and again, or perhaps anxiety as meetings approach.

Once you've spotted some of your own patterns, you can experiment with new responses that don't involve food but still offer relief. When stress starts to build or cravings pop up, try calling or texting a friend, even if it's just to say hi or vent for a minute. That bit of connection can be grounding. If you're restless or antsy, a five-minute walk (inside or out) can shift your energy and break the cycle of mindless munching. Engaging your hands with something creative, such as doodling on scrap paper, knitting a few rows, or tidying up a drawer, can satisfy the urge to do something without defaulting to food. Again, we aren't saying that you can never treat yourself to your favorite foods. But, instead, be aware of what you are eating and the reasons behind it.

THE PROFOUND EFFECTS OF VISUALIZATION

Visualization, also known as mental imagery or mental rehearsal, is the process of creating vivid, detailed images in the mind to simulate a desired outcome. Neuroscientific research shows that when we visualize an action, the brain activates many of the same neural pathways as it would if we were physically performing the task. For example, researchers at Harvard had a group of people play piano notes for five days and another group imagine they were playing notes. Both groups showed changes in the brain and millions of new neural connections (Hamilton 2012). This overlap helps the brain practice, improving performance, confidence, and even emotional regulation. Visualization works by enhancing focus, reducing anxiety, and priming the brain and body to respond more effectively in real situations. This practice can lower blood pressure, reduce pain, improve sleep, and speed up healing (St. James Rehabilitation & Healthcare Center 2025).

In psychology and performance coaching, visualization is widely used to help individuals achieve personal, athletic, and professional goals. Michael Phelps, the Olympic swimmer, used visualization extensively before his races, mentally rehearsing the races in detail, including the sound of the crowd and the feel of the water. Similarly, Serena Williams has spoken about visualizing the sensations of the movements as she plays (Perform 2024). Even Jim Carrey famously wrote himself a $10 million check for "acting services rendered" and visualized receiving it years before his breakthrough role in "Dumb and Dumber" (Santos 2023).

If you are struggling to get started, you can use the following script for your first visualization.

Take a deep breath in ... and slowly exhale. Let your body relax. Allow your shoulders to drop and your jaw to soften. Feel your body becoming calm and still. Now, picture yourself standing in a peaceful, natural place, perhaps a forest, a beach, or a sunny meadow. The air is fresh and clean. You feel completely safe and supported here. With each breath, imagine a gentle wave of light and warmth moving through your body, starting at the top of your head and slowly flowing down to your toes. This light represents health, strength, and balance. As it moves through you, it brings healing, energy, and calm. Now see yourself smiling, your body vibrant and strong.

Your mind is clear. You are at ease. You move with purpose, you rest when you need to, and you nourish yourself with care and love. Repeat silently, "I am calm. I am healthy. I am whole." Let this feeling of wellness settle deep within you. Take one more deep breath in ... and slowly exhale. When you're ready, gently bring your awareness back to the present moment, feeling refreshed and centered.

Visualization is not just wishful thinking. It's a structured, intentional practice grounded in neuroscience. Whether used in sports, public speaking, healing, or self-confidence, visualization helps align the mind and body toward a common goal. When paired with action and preparation, it becomes a powerful tool for transformation.

To sum up this chapter, stress will always be part of modern life, but it doesn't need to dictate your habits or leave you feeling powerless. By practicing quick strategies that work for you, being mindful, and exploring visualization, you can reduce the risk of many chronic conditions and lead a more enjoyable life. Next up, we'll look at how digital habits shape your mental clarity and energy, because wellness isn't just about food or movement but protecting your focus in a noisy world.

LIFE IS TOO SHORT FOR INEFFECTIVE DIETS AND EXCRUCIATING WORKOUTS

"Wellness encompasses a healthy body, a sound mind, and a tranquil spirit. Enjoy the journey as you strive for wellness."

— LAURETTE GAGNON BEAULIEU

Over the years, perhaps even decades, you have seen numerous wellness fads come and go. Like many, you probably started each one eagerly, waiting for promised results that never came. It's not to say that these trends don't deserve merit, as some have seen results, albeit temporary.

The problem with them is that they assume each individual body is the same and will, therefore, react in the same way. How can you compare the body of a 20-year-old female to that of a 60-year-old man? Hormones alone will affect results. However, it's overwhelmingly difficult to tailor a particular diet or workout to match your needs without the right information. You know better than anyone that the search for this information can leave you with more questions than answers.

That is until now. You have reached the halfway point of the Wellness Blueprint, and you are starting to appreciate the benefits of a personalized plan. We have taken the latest science and turned it into practical solutions for your body, mind, and soul—all without drastic measures. And it's still just the early days of your transformation.

Unfortunately, with health issues on the rise, not everyone is in the same position as you. There are so many people who are lost in a world of complex information when all they want to do is take control of their wellness. Although you may not realize it, there is a simple and small act you can do to help.

By leaving an honest review of this book on Amazon, others can see that answers are waiting for them and that they, too, can achieve amazing results in their health.

We understand that you're busy, so the process is straightforward and only takes a few minutes. Nevertheless, it's a few minutes that could make all the difference to the next person. Thank you in advance. Now, let's focus on your own wellness and explore the role of technology in your well-being.

Scan the QR code below

8

DIGITAL WELLNESS

Managing Tech for Mental Clarity

In some ways, technology is a little like stress. We can't live in this modern world without it, and in some cases, it can be useful, just like the right amount of stress can be motivating. But, there has come a point where we see people out for dinner all on their phones, or they go to sports events and concerts, spending more time videoing than appreciating the live performance. Nomophobia (no mobile phobia) is no longer a word to use lightly. A meta-analysis showed a prevalence of 94 percent, with one in five university students having moderate nomophobia and one in five a severe case (Al-Mamun 2025). The trick is, as with most of life, finding the right balance between using technology for its benefits and taking a break every now and then.

THE DIGITAL DETOX BLUEPRINT: UNPLUG WITHOUT FALLING BEHIND

You're texting in a group chat, your thumb aches, and notifications keep popping up—work email, memes, banking alerts. You promise yourself "just one more thing," but suddenly forty minutes have passed and your coffee's cold. This isn't about willpower. It's simply life in 2025. Nearly everything, from scheduling and catching up to relaxing, revolves around a screen. Tech is here to stay, and you need it, but all the buzzing and scrolling can leave you anxious, foggy, or disconnected. One study found that the excessive use of screens causes thinning of the cerebral cortex, the part of the brain responsible for decision-making, problem-solving, and processing memories (Descourouez 2024). This highlights the need for a digital detox.

Let's clear things up: a digital detox doesn't require a total tech black-out. You don't need to disappear from texts or miss deadlines to reset. Detoxing is about intentional breaks from technology to give your mind and body room to recharge, without abandoning your actual responsi-bilities. Think of it as a digital reset, flexible and tailored to your life. Maybe it's a few mindful, screen-free minutes, or a whole morning offline now and then. You pick what works.

Start small. Micro-detoxes are powerful. Try thirty minutes tech-free after dinner with no scrolling and no background TV. Maybe you'll notice an urge to check your phone within five minutes, but that's normal. Or try a notification-free lunch by silencing everything. Leave your phone out of reach and see what it's like to really taste your food or focus on conversation. If that's manageable, try a screen-free Saturday morning once a month. Read, go for a walk, cook, or enjoy letting your mind wander. Having fun things planned for your digital detox can help keep idle hands busy.

Interactive: Start Your Digital Detox Diary

Before your next tech break (even just thirty minutes), jot down how you feel—stressed, tired, scattered? After your unplugged time, write a few quick notes on any shifts. Perhaps it's a better mood, creativity, calm, or focus? Keep a digital detox diary for a week or two. You might spot patterns like your evenings get calmer, or mornings are smoother without an early scroll.

One reader told us she finally tried unplugging for a whole weekend after months of burnout from nonstop texts and emails. She feared missing something important, but ended up laughing more with her family and felt recharged for the week ahead. It wasn't about quitting tech. It was about using it on her own terms.

DESIGNING SCREEN BOUNDARIES: PROTECTING FOCUS AND SLEEP

Screen time messes with the brain in ways you might not even notice until you try to put your phone down. It's not just about feeling tired after a Netflix binge or zoning out during endless scrolling. We have seen how blue light, which pours from your phone, TV, and tablet, tells your brain it's daytime, even if it's midnight. Social media and news apps play another trick. Every like we get on social media causes a rush of dopamine, the feel-good hormone. Addiction expert Dr. Anna Lembke says our smartphones are creating dopamine junkies "with each swipe, like, and tweet feeding our habit" (Waters 2021).

Setting boundaries is about protecting what matters: focus, rest, and genuine presence. One easy place to start is with time-based boundaries. Try setting a clear "no screens" rule at the dinner table. Eating together without phones creates space for actual conversation and helps your brain switch out of work mode. If family or roommates push back, suggest an experiment: "Let's try thirty minutes without phones and see how it feels." Make it playful, a competition to see who can go longest without checking their device, or the first to check their phone pays for a round of drinks. Location-based boundaries work wonders, too. Charge your devices outside the bedroom. For example, leave your phone in the kitchen or hallway overnight. Use an old-school alarm clock if you need one. This simple change can transform your bedroom into a true sanctuary and protect your sleep from the blue light trap.

Activity-based boundaries offer another layer of protection for your attention. Install app timers for social media. Most modern phones let you set daily limits for Instagram, TikTok, or whatever eats up your time. You can set notifications for when you are getting close to your time limit or have apps automatically switch off (Unplugged, n.d.). You can also set deep work blocks during the day. Maybe it's just an hour or two when notifications are off and email is closed so you can actually think.

Home design can help too, even in small spaces. Try creating a screen-free sanctuary in your bedroom or a cozy corner of the living room. Keep books, journals, or puzzles within reach instead of remote controls or charging cords. Mornings are prime for analog rituals. Sip coffee while reading something on real paper or writing in a journal before touching your phone. If you live with others, use a family tech basket during meals when everyone tosses in their device before sitting down. It sounds simple, but collecting phones together signals that a real connection matters more than endless notifications.

Pushback is normal, especially if others are used to you being instantly reachable. Work emergencies can crop up, or maybe you're on call as a caregiver or parent. Flexibility helps here. If you're expecting something urgent, keep your phone on silent with vibration for specific contacts only. Let others know honestly, "I'm stepping away from screens for an hour but will check messages at 9 p.m." For those who resist family screen boundaries, keep the tone positive and low-pressure: "What if we try one meal a week with no devices?" If someone needs to be available for emergencies, like a doctor or parent of young kids, set rules together like "Phones face down unless we're waiting for an important call."

It's easy to break boundaries when you're tired, stressed, or just craving escape. If you find yourself sneaking extra screen time at night or during meals, pause and ask what you really need. Is it rest, connection, or distraction? Sometimes acknowledging what's behind the urge helps you swap scrolling for something that actually meets the need.

Boundaries aren't walls. They're flexible guardrails that help you protect your focus and sleep without cutting yourself off from work or loved ones. With each small adjustment, charging outside the bedroom, one tech-free meal a day, a little analog ritual in the morning, you create space for deeper rest and more meaningful attention throughout your day. If something doesn't work perfectly right away, adjust as needed.

MINDFUL TECH: USING DEVICES TO SUPPORT, NOT SABOTAGE, WELLNESS

Technology, often perceived as a barrier to wellness, can, in fact, be a powerful ally in cultivating healthy habits when used with intention. By selecting digital tools that align with personal wellness goals, individuals can transform their devices into instruments of health and growth. Meditation applications like Calm and Headspace offer pockets of tranquility amid chaos. Both enable you to tailor meditation practices (Osman 2024). Habit trackers such as Habitica and Streaks encourage goal setting and celebrate achievements. Habitica turns habit-building into games, and Streaks is ideal for building and maintaining habits (Guinness 2024). Setting reminders for hydration or movement can seamlessly integrate wellness into daily life, with gentle nudges from a device facilitating these habits. Gratitude apps encourage reflection on daily joys, promoting a positive mindset without the distraction of social validation. In essence, steering technology to serve wellness objectives empowers individuals to harness their devices as tools for personal development and well-being.

But tech can also create clutter, both digital and mental, if your phone feels crowded with apps you never use. It's normal for things to get messy, but what matters is how you reset. Start by taking a hard look at what's on your home screen. Scroll through every app and ask, "Do I use this? Does it add value?" If not, delete or archive it. For the ones you keep but don't need daily, move them off your main screen so they don't distract you. Silence notifications from apps that aren't urgent. Do you really need breaking news alerts at midnight? Probably not. Set limits on anything that tends to suck you in, like social media or shopping apps. Next, tackle your email inbox. Unsubscribe from newsletters or sales lists that do nothing but raise your stress level. You'll be amazed how much lighter you feel when only the important stuff remains.

Tech isn't just a tool for distraction. It's also a bridge for real connection and personal growth. Instead of falling into the trap of endless scrolling, use your devices to strengthen bonds with friends and family. Schedule a video call with someone you miss, even if it's just fifteen minutes on a random Tuesday. If you have a shared interest, like books, recipes, or hiking, join an online community focused on that topic. These groups can make you feel seen and supported in ways that scrolling through strangers' highlight reels never could. Podcasts and audiobooks are another great way to use tech for inspiration during commutes or chores. Try swapping out half an hour of social media for a podcast episode on something that fires up your creativity or teaches you a new skill. Suddenly, tech becomes an engine for learning and joy instead of just another source of noise.

One powerful habit is checking in with yourself about how tech makes you feel, not just what it helps you do. When you finish thirty minutes online, pause for a moment and notice whether you are more anxious. Drained? Maybe inspired or more connected? This self-reflection is key to shifting habits from autopilot to intention. Create a weekly ritual (Sunday evenings are great) to review your screen time stats and set intentions for the week ahead. Ask questions like: Did my phone time help me relax, learn, or connect? Or did it just make me restless? Adjust based on your answers, as there's no right or wrong here. It's about noticing patterns and making tweaks that serve you better.

A reader once told me she swapped her late-night phone scrolling for reading on an e-reader with warm backlighting, a small change that helped her wind down without the blue glow of her phone screen. Within a week, she noticed she was falling asleep faster and waking up less groggy. This is a great example of mindful swapping.

App Audit Checklist

- Which apps do I actually use every week?
- Which ones distract or stress me out?
- Which can I delete, silence, or move off my main screen?
- Are there subscriptions draining my wallet or focus?
- Which notifications can I turn off today?

Doing this once a season is like tidying up your digital closet. You clear out what doesn't fit and make room for what actually supports your goals.

Stepping back, tech is neither all good nor all bad. It's a tool, and how you use it shapes your well-being far more than any single device ever could. Whether it's turning reminders into little acts of self-care, curating your digital space like a home that welcomes calm, or connecting with people who lift you up, mindful tech puts the power back in your hands.

As we wrap up this chapter, remember that technology can help create clarity and connection when used with intention. The next chapter will explore how tracking progress and celebrating small wellness wins keeps motivation high and helps positive changes truly stick.

9

TRACKING PROGRESS

Celebrating Wins Beyond the Scale

There's something deeply satisfying about marking achievements, whether it's crossing off a list with a pen or marking something with a digital tick. That simple, physical action makes an accomplishment real, not just another unnoticed moment. Imagine if you could actually see your progress build up. Those little rushes of dopamine the brain rewards you with can be turned into something tangible!

THE WELLNESS WINS JAR: CAPTURING SMALL VICTORIES EVERY DAY

Enter the Wellness Wins Jar, a visual, tangible way to honor the seemingly minor, uncelebrated choices that truly add up to a healthier, happier you. The concept is simple: set out a jar, cup, or any container in a visible spot. Every time you make a choice that supports your well-being, drop in a note, marble, or bead. Maybe you pick water over soda, take five minutes of fresh air after work, or say no to a commitment you can't handle. Each action counts as a win. This physical act helps reinforce positive behavior and keep motivation strong, especially when progress feels invisible or self-criticism creeps in.

The magic isn't just in watching your wins accumulate but in the new mindset it nurtures. All-or-nothing thinking isn't the only cognitive distortion we are susceptible to. Negativity bias is a phenomenon whereby we tend to focus more on the negative than the positive. It's why it's easier for us to remember the criticism more than the compliments, the bad memories over the good ones, and the mistakes over the achievements. We even experience negative events more intensely. The negativity bias is closely linked to loss aversion, another cognitive distortion where the pain of loss is twice as powerful as the pleasure experienced when gaining something (Pilat et al., n.d.). The Wellness Wins Jar is an excellent visual reminder of the small positive moments that often get lost in the day. These micro-wins, over time, form the foundation of real change. They show that progress isn't always about dramatic transformations or big achievements. It's about consistently taking care of yourself in small ways.

Wins are personal and flexible. One day, just getting out of bed on time may feel like a triumph. Another day, it might be skipping dessert, an extra round of reps, or taking the stairs at work. This practice encourages you to look for successes across every part of wellness, not just nutrition and exercise, but also rest, boundaries, self-kindness, and even laughter. For some, saying "no" can be as significant as hitting a fitness goal.

Customize your wins jar or list however suits your life. For families, keep a communal jar in the kitchen and add slips during dinner. Kids and adults alike enjoy counting their wins and sharing them. It can encourage friendly encouragement or even a little competition. For roommates or partners, a shared jar can lead to mutual support and humor ("Good job resisting Karen's cupcakes!"). If you're often on the go or prefer digital tools, create a wins list in your phone's notes app. Jot down each win, even as a single word or emoji.

The real value comes from reviewing your wins. On tough days or when motivation dips, pull three slips from your jar and read them aloud, reminding yourself progress is happening, even if it's hard to see. At the end of each month, empty your jar and spread out all your notes. If you have gone for beads or marbles, sit with your jar and take a moment for reflection. Perhaps you can remember moments that the token represents. You might discover that the small, everyday victories mean the most. Sometimes that quick walk mattered more than a perfect gym session because it happened on a hard day.

Interactive Element: Building Your Own Wellness Wins Jar

Materials: Any jar, cup, bowl, pouch, or just your phone's notes app.

- **Step 1:** Place your container somewhere you'll see it often (kitchen counter, nightstand, desk).
- **Step 2:** Keep slips of paper, marbles, beads, or small tokens nearby.
- **Step 3:** Every time you make a positive wellness choice, big or small, add a token to your jar or log it in your app.
- **Step 4:** On difficult days, or monthly, review your wins, read three out loud, or share them with someone supportive.
- **Step 5:** Celebrate! Pick a win each month that made you proud, and note it somewhere special.

Over time, these tokens become living proof that meaningful change is already happening, one small win at a time.

MOOD, ENERGY, AND MINDFUL MINUTES: CREATIVE METRICS FOR SUCCESS

If you've ever stepped on a scale, waited for a number to change, and felt nothing but frustration, you're not alone. So many adults fall into the trap of thinking progress is only measured by pounds lost or the shape of their bodies. Yet, the real snapshots of health are often more subtle, like how steady your mood feels, how much pep you've got in your step, or how often you remember to take a slow breath in the midst of chaos. These are the signals that tell you whether your wellness habits are working for you behind the scenes. When you start paying attention to mood, energy, and mindful moments, you'll notice wins that numbers can't touch.

Mood is a powerful indicator of well-being. Your emotional state colors every part of your day. If you wake up hopeful, or at least neutral, tasks seem manageable, and even setbacks don't sting as much. Low moods, on the other hand, make everything harder, from work to home life and even self-care. Research points to the fact that our mood directly impacts our ability to stick with healthy changes over time; when you feel good, keeping up with habits becomes easier. An upbeat mental state has also been linked to lower blood pressure, healthier weight, better blood sugar levels, and less risk of heart disease (NIH, n.d.). That's why tracking how you feel, in plain language or with simple color codes, offers a more honest picture of your progress than any calorie count or clothing size.

Energy, your inner battery, works the same way. High-energy days are smoother. You breeze through tasks and find motivation to do things that seemed impossible yesterday. Low energy can feel like slogging through mud. Tracking your energy helps you see which habits give you a boost and what drains you dry. Maybe you spot patterns like feeling energized after a solid night's sleep and a walk before breakfast leads to your afternoon slump disappearing. Or perhaps too many late-night screens leave you dragging in the morning.

Mindful minutes round out this trio. These are any moments when you're truly present, whether you're sipping coffee without your phone in your hand, pausing to breathe during a tense meeting, or noticing the way sunlight hits your kitchen table. Mindful time doesn't have to mean meditation on a cushion. It's simply being where you are, even if just for sixty seconds. Tallying these mindful pauses brings awareness to how much space you're giving yourself to reset amid constant motion. The more mindful moments you collect, the easier it gets to break stress spirals and enjoy what's right in front of you.

Logging these metrics doesn't have to be another chore. You can keep things low-key and fun with analog tools. Try a mood color wheel where each day gets a shade, blue for calm, yellow for happy, red for stressed, and green for energized. Stick it on the fridge or in your planner as a visual mood map. For energy, sketch a simple sparkline in your journal, a line that rises and falls based on how charged or drained you feel each day. Some people like to use stickers or smiley faces, marking each page with quick feedback about how their body and brain showed up.

Digital options work well, too. Many phone apps let you log moods with emojis or short words. You can set reminders to check in at lunch or before bed: "How's my energy?" or "Did I pause today?" For mindful minutes, use tally marks on a sticky note or checkmarks in your calendar every time you carve out a moment to pay attention on purpose.

The real gold comes from reviewing these logs over time. At the end of each week, look back and ask yourself, "What boosted my energy most this week?" "Did my mood shift after I added a new habit?" Maybe increasing mindful minutes on Tuesday led to a calmer midweek, or skipping breakfast coincided with an energy dip by noon. These patterns help you adjust your routines based on what actually works, not just what you think should work.

Sometimes, these observations reveal surprises. A reader once told me she noticed her afternoon blues faded whenever she took three mindful minutes after lunch, even though nothing else changed about her diet or exercise routine. Another found that simply tracking moods helped him spot early signs of burnout before he crashed.

Visual reminders add a layer of motivation and pride. Try creating a wall chart with colored dots for each day's mood or energy level. Snap a photo of your mood wheel at the end of each week and share it with friends who understand what you're working toward. Even if you prefer to keep things private, these visual cues offer quiet encouragement when motivation dips. On rough days, looking back at your colorful logbook or looking through cheerful emojis reminds you that better days happen and will come again.

If tracking feels awkward at first, start small. Check in twice a week with one metric (mood or energy), then expand as it becomes routine. You'll find that noticing your own patterns builds self-trust and gives you permission to celebrate growth that no scale can measure. Mood, energy, and mindful minutes are proof that wellness is about living more fully, not just changing how you look.

HOW TO CELEBRATE YOUR WINS

Celebrating wellness wins, no matter how small, is a powerful way to reinforce progress and build long-term habits. Acknowledging milestones like getting better sleep, drinking more water, or managing stress more effectively boosts motivation and confidence. You don't need grand gestures to recognize your growth. Sometimes the smallest, most personal rewards are the most meaningful.

On a budget, consider simple but intentional ways to reward yourself. Treat yourself to a relaxing bath with essential oils or a cozy evening with your favorite book or playlist. You can also create a DIY at-home spa night or make a vision board to reflect on how far you've come and where you're headed. Why not opt for a new plant? One colleague of ours (who will remain nameless) considers a new sponge and cleaning product to be a celebration of a win. As you can see, what you class as a treat for your achievement is as personal as your Wellness Blueprint.

For social celebrations, invite friends or family to join you in a healthy meal, a group yoga session, or a casual wellness-themed picnic. You might host a small gathering where each person shares a recent win, physical, mental, or emotional, and offer support and encouragement. Celebrating together strengthens relationships and creates a positive environment where wellness becomes a shared journey.

Ultimately, the key is to pause and honor the effort. Whether it's sticking to a routine, overcoming a setback, or simply showing up for yourself on a tough day, every step counts. When you treat your wellness journey with respect and joy, it becomes easier to keep going, a pleasure far from the punishment of a traditional diet.

As this chapter wraps up, remember that tracking progress is about noticing all the ways you're moving forward, not just what's easy to measure. Whether you celebrate solo, with a buddy, or as part of a group, each win matters and deserves celebration. Next up, we'll explore how to take your Wellness Blueprint from ideas into daily action, making long-term change feel achievable for your real life.

10

REAL LIFE, REAL SOLUTIONS

Personalizing Your Blueprint

E ver look at someone else's organized planner or perfectly portioned meal and think, "That works for them, not me"? Maybe you've copied a friend's favorite fitness app or tried a celebrity's routine, only to abandon it when it clashed with your real life. The truth is, wellness isn't one-size-fits-all. It's much more like building your own sandwich, plenty of choices and only you know what's right for you. The goal isn't to follow a right formula but rather to find what fits your actual circumstances right now. That's what the Adaptive Wellness Framework offers: a toolkit for making decisions, filtering options, and building a guilt-free, custom plan.

THE ADAPTIVE WELLNESS FRAMEWORK: CHOOSING WHAT WORKS FOR YOU

What sets this framework apart? You're in control. Instead of wondering, "What should I be doing?" you start with, "What do I need, want, and have capacity for?" The Adaptive Wellness Framework focuses on your unique needs and preferences so you can select strategies that fit your context. Imagine a plan that is built around your constraints and motivators, such as when you have energy, your budget, and your work schedule. This isn't about willpower. It's about smart choices that set you up for genuine success.

Think about it: If you're choosing between evening walks and morning yoga, the old advice might urge you to win the morning. But the Adaptive Wellness Framework suggests you move when your body prefers it. Maybe that's evening walks, since your mornings are usually rushed. Perhaps you are feeling extra stressed after a long day, and an evening yoga session will meet the needs of your mind and body. Or maybe you like variety, so you alternate. The point is to tailor your plan to your natural rhythms, skipping the shame or pressure of someone else's rules.

Start with a self-inventory. Take a notebook or your phone and answer these: What are your biggest barriers—time, energy, money, motivation, mobility? Which wellness area needs the most help right now? Nutrition, movement, sleep, or mindset? Be honest. Maybe money is tight or mornings are crazy. Maybe motivation is low, or sleep needs attention. Circle your top two challenges that feel most urgent.

Then, reflect:

- What truly motivates you?
- Do you want energy for work, to enjoy time with your kids, to feel more upbeat, or to be less stressed?
- What are your nonnegotiables—family dinners, weekend rest?
- What activities do you enjoy doing in your free time?
- Is there a habit you would like to kick?

This assessment isn't about blaming shortcomings but clarifying what matters so you can focus your energy effectively.

Now, the key shift: Adaptation always beats rigid rules. Life throws curveballs—work emergencies, switched moods, or missed grocery runs. Sometimes you swap fresh veggies for frozen or skip the gym in favor of stretching at home. The Adaptive Wellness Framework embraces these swaps. If your plan says thirty minutes of cardio but you grab three ten-minute walks between meetings, that's still progress. If Sunday's fresh meal prep turns into frozen stir-fry kits by midweek, that flexibility helps you stay on course, not stressed out.

Last year, we met Arthur, a retiree who felt isolated after leaving work. Rather than forcing intense workouts, Arthur made social connections his wellness anchor, joining a weekly walking group and hosting neighbors for tea. For him, movement meant connection over cardio, and his plan focused on relationships and gentle activity, not just step counts.

Interactive Element: Build Your Adaptive Wellness Map

Draw a decision tree. At the top, write your main wellness goal. Branch out with options based on your self-inventory, like evening energy or budget meal prep. Under each branch, jot down one or two strategies, such as evening walks with music or Sunday batch cooking with frozen veggies. Add backup plans for chaotic days, like a home workout video if it's raining or overnight oats if mornings are rushed. Put this map somewhere visible as a reminder of your flexible, adaptive approach.

The Adaptive Wellness Framework gives you permission to pick what works and to change it up as needed. By letting go of rigid systems and embracing personalization, you're building a realistic blueprint that evolves with you, not just for today but as life changes moving forward.

WELLNESS FOR SHIFT WORKERS, PARENTS, AND CAREGIVERS

If you are up past midnight, prepping for the next day, or finishing a late shift while the rest of the world sleeps, you know wellness can feel like a moving target. There's nothing quite like the life of a shift worker, parent, or caregiver. Schedules are all over the place. Sleep comes in fragments. You might eat lunch at 10 p.m., and your morning could start after sunset. The advice you see online, those tidy routines and sunrise yoga sessions, rarely match your reality. It's easy to feel dismissed, like wellness is reserved for people with open calendars and full nights of sleep. But your well-being matters just as much, maybe even more.

Take Lara, a nurse who alternates between day and night shifts every week. She explained to us that some mornings, she's making breakfast for her kids. Other days, she's winding down at sunrise after twelve hours on her feet. Her energy swings wildly, and she often finds herself grabbing whatever food is easy. She wishes she could follow the advice in those glossy wellness books, but her world is unpredictable. After we introduced her to the Adaptive Wellness Plan, she stopped comparing herself to what others were doing and focused on what she needed. She realized that in order to keep up with her irregular responsibilities, her priority was to stabilize her energy levels. Once she had mastered this, she found she had better mental clarity, and this enabled her to plan ahead for busy weeks with batch cooking, which, in turn, freed up more time for her to start an exercise routine.

You deserve wellness strategies that flex with your life, not rigid routines that leave you feeling guilty for missing some imaginary standard. For shift workers, meal prepping becomes an act of survival, not just convenience. Instead of planning for one big session each week, try split shift prepping. Chop veggies or portion snacks during brief windows between shifts or while kids watch a favorite show. Stack your fridge with grab-and-go foods like hard-boiled eggs, yogurt, cut fruit, and wraps so you're not left hungry and rushing for takeout when time runs short. If hot meals feel impossible during off-hours, breakfast-for-dinner or simple grain bowls can save you in a pinch.

Movement doesn't need to look traditional either. Five minutes is enough to wake up tired muscles or shake off stress after a long stretch at a desk or bedside. Turn movement into a game with your family. After dinner, toss on music and do a freeze dance, or challenge your kids to see who can do the funniest animal walk around the living room. These bursts keep you active while inviting laughter and connection, which can be just as restorative as exercise itself.

Most important for anyone juggling competing demands is letting go of the idea that wellness must be all or nothing. Good enough counts. If you only have three minutes to breathe deeply before the next task calls, take them. A parent once told us she did mindful breathing exercises while her toddler napped on her chest. Not fancy, but real—and it worked. A shift worker we know adjusted her routine by sleeping with eye masks and investing in blackout curtains. She also allowed herself to snack on frozen fruit instead of stressing over fresh produce every week.

Accountability helps, too. Try a buddy system where you check in with another parent, shift worker, or caregiver about daily wins or struggles. Celebrate when you squeeze in those micro-actions, a glass of water between diaper changes, a stretch during a short break, or a laugh shared after a long day. These wins add up and build resilience over time.

If resources are tight or time feels like it's always running out, remember that perfection isn't part of the equation here. Wellness can still include quick, nutritious meals eaten with one hand while holding a baby or gentle stretches done in scrubs before clocking in for the night shift. What matters is finding what works for now and giving yourself credit for showing up, even if it's only in small ways today.

NAVIGATING CHRONIC CONDITIONS AND LIMITATIONS: CUSTOMIZING WITH CONFIDENCE

The pervasive frustration stemming from wellness routines that fail to accommodate individual bodies and realities is palpable. For those living with chronic conditions or physical limitations, the deluge of generic advice isn't just ineffective—it's isolating. Attempts to adhere to "one-size-fits-all" plans often end in discouragement, not due to a lack of motivation, but because these needs are uniquely different. The wellness industry frequently overlooks the nuances of pain, fatigue, and medical constraints, making it seem as though some are merely spectators in their own health. However, every individual's health is valid and deserves recognition and support, regardless of the challenges faced.

Customization is not a weakness but a sign of resourcefulness and self-respect. Picture a reader named Tara, who has lived with arthritis for years. She once felt guilty about skipping high-impact workouts, but after some trial and error, she found that gentle movement routines in a chair allowed her to stretch and strengthen without flare-ups. She swapped out shame for curiosity, asking, "What feels good today?" rather than "What should I be doing?" That shift changed everything. It's natural to feel angry or sad about things your body struggles with.

Sometimes you might grieve the loss of ease or strength you once had. Allow those feelings, but don't let them convince you that wellness isn't for you.

Now, when you're thinking about starting something new, it's important to work with, not against, your medical realities. This doesn't mean giving up control. It means teaming up with your healthcare providers to build a plan that supports you safely. Next time you see your doctor, physical therapist, or dietitian, bring specific questions:

- Are there movements I should avoid?
- How can I adapt my nutrition for my diagnosis?
- What warning signs should I watch for?
- Is there a way to track progress that fits my abilities?
- Are there alternative medicines that can help manage my symptoms?

There's no need to memorize everything on the spot. For example, if you're managing diabetes, it's wise to track your meals. Your provider might help you tailor meal timing and carb choices to keep blood sugar steady while still eating foods you love.

Safe adaptation is not about doing less. It's about doing differently. If getting up and down from the floor is tough, seated routines or water-based activities may feel much better. There are entire yoga flows designed for chair practice so you can stretch and breathe fully without pain. Despite being seated, chair yoga still releases pain and tension, increases flexibility, stability, and strength, and reduces stress (Lomer 2023). If swallowing is an issue or chewing is hard, try softer textures like smoothies with nut butter or mashed sweet potatoes. Blended soups can also be delicious and nourishing. Chronic pain often flares unpredictably; on those days, restorative yoga poses or even gentle breathwork may be all you can manage, and that counts.

Don't be afraid to get creative with self-care. If standing in the kitchen leaves you exhausted, prep snacks while sitting down. Use assistive tools if needed—jar openers, reachers, or adaptive utensils can make meal prep less taxing. For movement, consider resistance bands instead of weights if your grip strength varies. Sometimes, technology is your ally. Audiobooks for guided meditation, voice-activated reminders for medication or hydration, and virtual support groups can keep you connected and encouraged.

We are always inspired by people who rewrite the rules to fit their bodies. One reader, living with multiple sclerosis, learned to conserve energy by habit stacking, pairing stretches with morning coffee or brief mindfulness breaks after checking emails. These micro-actions added up over time without draining her reserves. Another person who is blind shared how she uses podcasts and audio fitness guides to stay active. She's built a rich routine using sound as her primary tool.

Checklist: Questions for Your Healthcare Team

- Which types of activity are safest for me?
- Are there red flags I should watch for during exercise?
- How should I adjust my nutrition for my condition?
- Are there any medications or treatments that affect my energy or appetite?
- Can I track progress in ways beyond weight or steps?

Wellness becomes powerful when it meets you where you are, flexible enough to adapt yet strong enough to support growth. Your blueprint might look different from anyone else's, but it's just as valuable. Living with a chronic condition doesn't put up a stop sign. It just asks for a detour that honors both your boundaries and your dreams.

As this chapter closes, remember that personalizing wellness isn't just allowed; it's necessary. Every adjustment and creative workaround is a mark of wisdom. Your health story is worth writing in your own words. In the following chapter, we'll explore how resilience and motivation carry you forward when life gets unpredictable. Because every blueprint faces storms, and yours will weather them just fine.

11

MOTIVATION AND BOUNCE-BACK

Resilience After Setbacks

Ever notice how losing momentum sneaks up on you? One minute, you're feeling good, plugging away at your wellness plans, and the next, everything feels off. Maybe your workouts start slipping. Maybe your meal prep routine falls apart. Or you just wake up and realize all your healthy habits are buried under a pile of stress, work, and real-life chaos. It's like when you're driving and suddenly miss an exit, not because you meant to, but because your mind wandered or traffic was heavy. You don't pull over and give up on the trip. Your GPS doesn't scold you for messing up. It simply recalculates and suggests a new way forward. That's exactly what recalibration is all about.

THE POWER OF RECALIBRATION: WHAT TO DO WHEN YOU LOSE MOMENTUM

Recalibration is not starting from scratch or throwing away everything you've built. It's about pausing, taking stock, and shifting direction based on where you are right now, not where you thought you'd be or where you tell yourself you should be. It's an active choice to adjust your route. This mindset can be freeing because it lets you drop perfectionism and get creative instead. You're honoring your progress by learning and adapting. Think of recalibration as your own personal rerouting system, always ready to help you get back on track without shame, just a new map.

When momentum falters, identifying the root cause is vital. This could stem from clear disruptions, such as a family crisis, work overload, or health issues. Often, however, the triggers are subtler: dwindling motivation, ennui, overly ambitious goals, or shifts in daily life that disrupt established routines. Conducting a self-audit can reveal underlying issues. Consider whether your goals were unrealistic, changes in your life like a new job or relocation occurred, or if feelings of inspiration have been replaced by burnout. Documenting and honestly responding to these inquiries can highlight previously unnoticed patterns, helping you recognize changes in what motivates you and whether your surroundings support your desired habits.

Interactive Element: Self-Inventory Recalibration Journal

Grab your journal or phone. Give yourself space to reflect, not just on what went wrong, but on what's different now.

- What was my original goal or habit?
- When did I first notice things slipping?
- What has changed in my routine, energy, motivation, or environment?
- Was my goal so ambitious that it started feeling impossible?
- Did I lose interest because it got boring or too predictable?
- Did something external (workload, family needs, stress) shift unexpectedly?
- What parts of my routine still feel good? Which parts feel heavy or stressful?

Sometimes, the answers don't just pop out at you. If you can't put your finger on the answer straight away, it's worth using the Five Whys method. This is a method that helps you understand the cause and effect of a problem and get to the real root of it (Stanley 2019). It's simple, let's say you have stopped your morning workouts because you are waking up groggy; ask yourself why. Perhaps it's because you have been going to bed later, again, why? From here, you may discover that you have broken your own rules and been checking your emails a little later. Once again, why? The method says five whys, but in reality, you can use as many as you need until you get that light bulb moment and your setback makes sense. Once you've sorted out the why, it's time to pause, learn, recalibrate, and re-engage. This four-step process helps you move forward with less drama and more self-respect.

- **Step 1:** Pause. Give yourself permission to stop pushing for a moment. Don't beat yourself up; don't rush to fix everything overnight. Just acknowledge where you are without judgment or guilt. This is your reset button.
- **Step 2:** Learn. Look back at what was working before things stalled (even if only for a short while). What did you enjoy? What felt easy? Then get real about what didn't work. Was it too much, too repetitive, or did it clash with something else in your life? This is where honest reflection pays off.
- **Step 3:** Recalibrate. Adjust your plan based on what you've just discovered. Maybe you make your goal smaller or tweak your schedule so it actually matches your current life. Perhaps you swap out a boring workout for something new or change meal prep day because weekends are now packed with family stuff. The point isn't to lower your standards. It's to create a plan that feels possible right now.
- **Step 4:** Re-engage. Take one simple action, no matter how tiny, to get moving again. Maybe that's making your shower more mindful, a piece of fruit with your morning coffee, or walking to the corner store instead of driving. Regardless of the action you choose, make it achievable.

Let us share a couple of stories from readers who put recalibration into practice. One reader was always trying to fit in evening workouts but found her energy tanked after dinner. So she decided to switch her exercise to the morning, before work, starting with just fifteen minutes every other day. The change didn't require more effort. It simply matched her natural rhythms better. Another person loved elaborate meal plans, at first, but soon felt overwhelmed by recipes with too many steps and exotic ingredients. Instead of giving up on healthy eating altogether, he simplified his meals to basic mix-and-match bowls with familiar foods that were easier to find, which helped him stay consistent even during busy weeks.

When you treat recalibration as an expected part of growth and not as evidence of failure, you put yourself in the driver's seat again. Life will always be full of challenges, but your power lies in responding with flexibility instead of frustration.

THE BOUNCE-BACK PLAN: TURNING SETBACKS INTO SPRINGBOARDS

Setbacks can serve as your greatest teachers if you let them. Think of setbacks as data points, not final grades. Studies in behavioral psychology back this up. Often, folks who stumble and reflect make more lasting progress than those who expect a flawless run from day one. But this depends on the type of reflection. Replaying a situation isn't enough. In order to learn, you have to dig a little deeper (Maurer 2022). This requires a change in your thought patterns. We need to switch from this replaying, which often only leads to negative self-talk, and replace it with a learning mindset.

Instead of seeing the occasional flop as a reason to quit, build yourself a bounce-back plan. This plan is about pulling a lesson from the wreckage and using that lesson as fuel for your next step. The first move is simple but powerful: Acknowledge the setback without blame. Say it out loud or write it down, for example, "I missed my workouts last week," "I stress-ate after that meeting," or "I totally checked out on my sleep routine." Drop the need to assign fault. Guilt and blame are heavy, and they keep you stuck. Acceptance frees up mental space to figure out what's next.

After you've accepted what happened, draw on that experience for one clear insight. What's the single biggest thing this setback is trying to show you? The point isn't to create a laundry list of everything you did wrong. It's to find one thread worth pulling—a lesson that feels honest and actionable. Let's say you noticed that you never quite finished everything on your to-do lists, and in the end, you felt that there was no point in making these lists, then productivity started to slow down, and things got forgotten. You aren't going to learn anything if you simply replay all the things you didn't get around to doing. You are just going to feel bad about yourself. One possible lesson to learn from this is that you are an overachiever and set your expectations too high. From here, you can start from fresh, a new to-do list that keeps things realistic. This might involve just starting with two or three things on your list and then gradually adding to it each day until you find the sweet spot between a challenge and unrealistic expectations of yourself.

Whatever action you need to take, keep it visible and tangible. If movement slips, put your sneakers by the door tonight or text a friend to meet for a walk in the morning. When your eating habits fall apart, prep one healthy snack and put it front and center in the fridge. These actions are gentle reminders that change is possible right now, not later.

Real-life examples illustrate the adaptability of our wellness plan. One individual found that she had plateaued with her yoga routines and wasn't feeling the same benefits. She told us how frustrated she was with herself because she felt like she was a quitter when she stopped her classes. Then, she came across Pilates, and after the first class, she felt her joy and enthusiasm return. Similarly, another person tackled nightly snacking by identifying the root cause with the help of the Five Whys method. He shared with us that his loneliness was causing him to reach for the snack as a source of comfort. He shifted to healthier coping mechanisms, such as texting a friend or engaging in reading, instead of heading to the pantry. These adjustments underscore the importance of personalized strategies in achieving wellness.

You'll face moments when guilt, self-doubt, or even outside criticism try to drag you down after a setback. That's when bounce-back scripts come in handy, simple phrases you can keep on repeat until they start sinking in. You might want to try, "This is a chance to learn, not a reason to quit." Or maybe, "Every wellness plan has detours. Mine is still underway." These aren't cheesy affirmations. They're reminders that progress is made in fits and starts.

People find creative ways to turn setbacks into momentum all the time. One reader started keeping a gratitude log after weeks of feeling negative and burned out at work. She noticed her mood slowly shift just by writing down three things she appreciated each night. Another parent realized meal prep had totally fallen apart (again), but instead of giving up, he invited his kids into the kitchen for build-your-own dinner nights. He sent us an email saying family meals had become less stressful and something everyone looked forward to.

The truth is, bouncing back isn't about having superhuman discipline or never making mistakes. It's about seeing setbacks as springboards, opportunities to adjust, learn, and move forward with new tools in your pocket. Each time you bounce back, you build resilience muscles that make it easier next time life throws you off balance. You'll start to notice the bounce-back gets faster, your goals become more flexible, and your confidence grows with each comeback.

FINAL TIPS FOR MOTIVATION AND RESILIENCE

Let's begin by exploring motivation on a deeper level. There are two main types: intrinsic and extrinsic motivation. Intrinsic motivation comes from within, doing something because it's personally rewarding or aligned with your values. For example, choosing to exercise because it makes you feel energized and mentally clear is an intrinsic motivator. In contrast, extrinsic motivation comes from outside sources, like working out to lose weight for a vacation or because a doctor recommends it (Indeed 2025). Both types can be effective, but intrinsic motivation is generally more sustainable over time.

When it comes to wellness, understanding what motivates you can help you stay on track. People often start with extrinsic goals, such as fitting into a certain size or earning praise. However, lasting wellness is more likely when you find deeper, internal reasons for making healthy choices. This might include wanting to feel stronger, be a role model for your children, or manage stress more effectively. Building habits that are meaningful and enjoyable increases the likelihood that you'll stick with them. Reflecting on your personal "why" and shifting your mindset from "I have to" to "I choose to" can transform motivation into a long-term lifestyle change.

Motivation and resilience are closely linked because both play a vital role in how we respond to challenges, setbacks, and long-term goals, especially with regard to wellness. Motivation gives us the reason to start taking action, while resilience helps us keep going when things get tough. For example, if someone is motivated to improve their health, they might begin exercising or eating more mindfully. But when obstacles arise, like fatigue, a busy schedule, or a plateau in progress, it's resilience that allows them to stay committed and bounce back rather than give up. In this way, resilience acts like a support system for motivation, especially when willpower alone isn't enough (Ademusoyo 2025).

At the same time, motivation can fuel resilience. When you have a strong internal reason or clear goal, you're more likely to keep pushing through discomfort or setbacks. Intrinsic motivation, such as a desire to feel better mentally or live longer for your family, can give you a deeper well of emotional strength to draw from when challenges arise. Together, motivation and resilience create a powerful combination for long-term growth, healthy habits, and personal change.

Everything that we have looked at in this chapter so far can help you build resilience, but there are three more strategies that can make a powerful difference: self-awareness, emotional regulation, and cognitive reframing.

Self-awareness and emotional regulation are foundational components of resilience, particularly in how we respond to stress, adversity, and emotional discomfort. Self-awareness is the ability to recognize and understand your own thoughts, emotions, and behavioral patterns in real time (Warley 2025). When someone is self-aware, they can catch the early signs of emotional overwhelm, like frustration, anxiety, or hopelessness, before these feelings spiral out of control. This awareness allows for a more thoughtful and constructive response rather than a reactive one.

Emotional regulation builds on this by enabling individuals to manage their emotional responses in ways that support long-term well-being.

Instead of suppressing emotions, regulation involves acknowledging them, understanding their root causes, and choosing appropriate coping strategies, such as breathing exercises, reframing negative thoughts, or seeking support, instead of reacting in negative ways (McGarvie 2025). Together, self-awareness and emotional regulation help build resilience by reducing impulsive reactions, preventing burnout, and maintaining a clear sense of purpose and perspective during difficult times. In the context of wellness, these skills can make the difference between giving up after a setback and adapting constructively, ultimately supporting a more sustainable and compassionate journey toward health and growth.

Finally, at its core, cognitive reframing involves consciously shifting the way you perceive a situation in order to view it in a more constructive or empowering light. For example, instead of seeing a missed workout as a failure, a reframed perspective might view it as a needed rest day or an opportunity to reassess one's routine. This doesn't mean ignoring difficulties or pretending everything is positive, as this comes dangerously close to toxic positivity. Toxic positivity is the excessive and ineffective overgeneralization of a happy, optimistic state across all situations, even when it's not appropriate. It involves dismissing or minimizing genuine emotional experiences by insisting on a positive outlook, no matter how difficult things are. For example, telling someone who recently lost their job to "just stay positive" or "everything happens for a reason" can invalidate their grief or frustration (Insights Psychology 2025). Instead, cognitive reframing is about choosing interpretations that support growth, motivation, and psychological flexibility.

In the context of wellness, reframing helps break the cycle of negative self-talk that often leads to guilt, shame, or giving up. It encourages individuals to see setbacks as part of the process rather than as permanent defeats. Cognitive reframing helps remove cognitive distortions and create helpful thoughts that are based on evidence (Mohn 2024). In the past, you may have told yourself, "I missed two workouts this week. I'm a failure." There is no evidence that proves you are a failure because there is still time to succeed. A more beneficial thought would be "Missing two workouts doesn't erase my progress. I've been making healthier choices, and I can start again tomorrow." Over time, this mindset strengthens emotional resilience by reinforcing the belief that health and well-being are ongoing journeys, not all-or-nothing endeavors. By practicing cognitive reframing regularly, individuals become better equipped to navigate stress, adapt to change, and stay committed to their goals, even in the face of obstacles.

As we close this chapter on motivation and bouncing back, take a moment to think about a situation where you faced a challenge and came through it with resilience. It doesn't have to be related to your well-being. Perhaps you had a difficult client to work with or a toddler's temper tantrum in the middle of a grocery store? Each obstacle you have overcome is a reminder that you can do the same when it comes to your wellness plan. Fortunately, there is still plenty more to add to your plan, and in the next chapter, we are going to discover more about your vagus nerve and how this relates to the mind-body connection.

12

THE MIND-BODY CONNECTION

Holistic Wellness in Action

Imagine you're stuck in traffic on a gray Monday, tapping the steering wheel and trying not to lose your cool. Your jaw clenches, your stomach flips, and soon a headache starts. Tension lingers even when you try to relax. This isn't stress just in your head. It's in your muscles, gut, and even your skin. Thoughts and emotions ripple through every system in your body, and your body fires signals right back, influencing your mind in return. This feedback loop is real, and it affects how you feel, move, and act every single day.

THE MIND-BODY LOOP: HOW THOUGHTS, EMOTIONS, AND HEALTH INTERACT

We need a little science to fully appreciate the mind-body connection. Let's have a quick review of the stress response. When stress or emotions like anger or worry hit, your brain launches a cascade of responses. Neurotransmitters are chemical messengers that race through neural pathways. The hypothalamus triggers the release of adrenaline, which kick-starts the "fight-or-flight" response, and noradrenaline, which affects blood pressure, heart rate, and focus (Cleveland Clinic 2022b). Stress can even impact your cells.

But the flow goes both ways: your physical state shapes your mindset right back. When you're sleep-deprived, your mind feels foggy, and it's tough to make good decisions. Pain or low energy can cause frustration, fuel negative thoughts, and eat away at motivation. Even small physical issues like muscle aches or a sluggish gut can erode patience and confidence. That's why a restless night often leads to snapping at loved ones or doubting yourself at work.

These cycles build on themselves. For instance, worrying about a deadline might keep you up at night. Without enough sleep, you wake up groggy and irritable, with low patience and concentration. Every small obstacle now feels huge. This can spark more worry or physical symptoms like headaches, fueling the loop all over again. Researchers call these feedback loops, where each part strengthens the next, making it tough to break free unless you notice it happening (Lumen Learning, n.d.). It's clear to see how tension in the muscles can be caused by stress, but this doesn't explain how, for example, you get butterflies in your stomach when you are nervous. The answer lies in your vagus nerve.

The brain-gut axis is the complex communication network that links the central nervous system (CNS) with the enteric nervous system (ENS) in the gastrointestinal tract. One of the most important components of this system is the vagus nerve, which serves as a key highway transmitting signals between the brain and the gut. This two-way communication allows the brain to influence gut function (like digestion and motility) and, conversely, allows the gut to send information about its state back to the brain. The vagus nerve plays a vital role in regulating inflammation, mood, and stress responses. Research has shown that a healthy gut microbiome can positively influence mental health by sending calming signals to the brain through the vagus nerve, while chronic stress or poor diet can disrupt this connection, potentially contributing to anxiety, depression, or digestive issues (Han et al. 2022).

So, how can you interrupt those negative loops before they spiral? It starts by spotting early warning signs. With practice, this gets easier. Notice if your shoulders are tensed, your jaw is clenched, or negative thoughts keep repeating. When you catch yourself in the cycle, use the "Name it to Tame it" technique. Pause, then label the emotion, for example, "I'm feeling anxious," or "I am angry." Naming emotions pulls them out of autopilot and gives you a bit of space to respond. Neuroscience studies have proven that saying the intense emotion aloud or in your head turns the emotion into language and reduces activity in the amygdala. Other research shows that labeling your emotions increases activity in the prefrontal lobe, the part of the brain responsible for logic, reason, and rational thinking (Anxiety NZ, n.d.). It sounds too simple to be that effective, but the science backing this technique makes it an invaluable tool to try.

To reduce the likelihood of negative loops, it's important that we feed the brain-gut axis with the right foods. The brain-gut axis thrives on a balanced and diverse gut microbiome, which directly influences mental and physical health. Our gut contains about 100 million neurons, often referred to as the "second brain." This network of neurons allows the gut to communicate closely with the brain, largely via the vagus nerve. Remarkably, the gut is responsible for producing approximately 95 percent of the body's serotonin, a neurotransmitter that plays a critical role in regulating mood, sleep, and appetite (Appleton 2018). A well-nourished gut microbiome helps regulate this serotonin production, supporting emotional well-being and cognitive function.

To nourish the gut-brain axis, it's essential to include both probiotics and prebiotics in the diet. Probiotics are live beneficial bacteria found in foods like yogurt, kefir, sauerkraut, kimchi, and miso. These help maintain and restore the balance of good bacteria in the gut. Prebiotics, on the other hand, are nondigestible fibers that serve as food for these good bacteria. They are found in foods such as garlic, onions, leeks, asparagus, bananas, and oats. Together, probiotics and prebiotics help reduce inflammation, support immune function, and improve the production of neurotransmitters like serotonin. Regular consumption of these gut-supporting nutrients can enhance mental clarity, reduce symptoms of anxiety or depression, and contribute to overall wellness by optimizing the function of the brain-gut axis (Harvard Health Publishing 2022).

Interactive Element: Interrupting the Loop

Try to get into the habit of consuming probiotics and prebiotics on a daily basis. Aside from this, pick one of these habits and use it the next time you feel stressed:

- Label your intense emotions aloud or in your head.
- Remind yourself that this moment will pass.
- Stand, stretch overhead, and shake out your arms for twenty seconds.
- Step outside and walk for five minutes—even just around the block.
- Use cognitive reframing for negative thoughts.

Once you begin breaking negative cycles, you can also build up positive ones, which we call wellness snowballs. After a morning workout, even a short one, notice what you're grateful for, maybe just that you got moving at all. That mood boost can help you make better food choices or handle stress later. Or, notice how focused you feel after eating mindfully. Link that clarity to an affirmation like "I support my body with good choices." These small wins build momentum, creating upward spirals of confidence and energy.

It doesn't require dramatic changes. Any time you feel even a little better after moving, pausing, or being kind to yourself, celebrate it, even just mentally. Over time, these positive moments can add up, helping healthy feedback loops become the norm rather than the rare exception.

BREATHWORK AND BODY AWARENESS: SIMPLE TOOLS FOR EVERYDAY CALM

Your body often seems in control, particularly during stress-induced moments when your chest tightens or anxiety quickens your breath. Yet, many overlook the power of conscious breathing in regaining control. Breathwork is accessible to all and at any moment. Previously, you may have thought this was just giving you some recycled advice, but now that you are aware of the science (breathwork to stimulate the vagus nerve), it's time to look at other techniques apart from box breathing.

The simplest version is a deep inhale through your nose, filling your lungs until your belly rises, then an even slower exhale through pursed lips. But if you want a little more structure (and maybe a better shot at sticking with it), try these three techniques and see which clicks for you. For winding down before sleep or after a restless day, the "4-7-8" breath is a gentle favorite. Breathe in quietly through your nose for a count of four, hold that breath for seven counts (don't stress if you can't reach seven at first), then let it out for eight counts (Fletcher 2024). Repeat this cycle four times and notice if your muscles unclench or your mind gets quieter.

Alternate nostril breathing is a yogic practice and a powerful breath control technique used to calm the nervous system and balance the mind. This practice involves inhaling through one nostril while closing the other with a finger, then switching nostrils for the exhale, and repeating the cycle in a rhythmic pattern. Scientifically, alternate nostril breathing has been shown to reduce stress, lower heart rate, and support autonomic nervous system balance, especially by stimulating the parasympathetic nervous system. It also helps to regulate the flow of oxygen to both hemispheres of the brain, improving focus, clarity, and emotional regulation. Practicing this technique for just a few minutes daily can enhance resilience, reduce anxiety, and support overall mental and physical well-being (Gilbert 2024).

Coherent breathing, also known as resonant breathing, promotes balance between the mind and body by slowing the breath to approximately five to six breaths per minute. This practice typically involves inhaling through the nose for a count of five or six seconds and then exhaling for the same count, creating a smooth, rhythmic cycle. Coherent breathing stimulates the parasympathetic nervous system and also improves heart rate variability (HRV), a key marker of nervous system health, which reflects the body's ability to adapt to stress (Mind Mics 2023). When you align breath with the body's natural rhythms, coherent breathing encourages a deeper mind-body connection, encouraging a state of calm awareness and inner balance that supports both mental and physical well-being.

Breathwork gets even more powerful when paired with body awareness. Most of us live from the neck up all day, forgetting we even have bodies until something hurts or aches. Tuning into physical sensations on purpose can ground you and teach you how to spot tension or emotional build-up before it spills into headaches or fatigue. Progressive Muscle Relaxation (PMR) strengthens the mind-body connection by teaching you to recognize and release physical tension. Developed by Dr. Edmund Jacobson in the early twentieth century, PMR involves systematically tensing and then relaxing specific muscle groups, typically starting from the feet and working up to the head. For example, you might begin by tightly squeezing your toes for a few seconds, then slowly releasing and noticing the sensation of relaxation. This process is repeated through each major muscle group. Practicing PMR helps bring awareness to where you hold tension, often unconsciously, and provides a practical method to let it go (Komoder 2024). PMR enhances the mind-body connection by shifting attention inward, grounding you in the present moment. Over time, it trains the brain to associate physical relaxation with mental calm, which is especially beneficial for those dealing with stress, chronic pain, or high emotional reactivity.

Movement can be just as mindful as stillness. Next time you walk, whether down a hallway or through the grocery store, try focusing on each step, the heel touching down, weight rolling forward, or toes lifting off. Notice how arms swing, how breath flows in and out of your nose. If thoughts wander, gently bring them back to the rhythm of walking. This simple act can shift your mood and help reset a busy mind. Combine mindful walking with the 5-4-3-2-1 grounding technique to fully engage your senses and your mind.

Integrating these tools into daily life doesn't require extra time carved out of an already packed schedule. Instead, tuck them into routines you already have. Before opening an email in the morning or at work, pause for five to six slow breaths before diving in. Waiting for water to boil or riding an elevator? Try box breathing. Before meals or meetings, take a grounding breath: inhale deeply, feel your feet on the floor, and exhale slowly while relaxing your jaw and shoulders. Even during difficult conversations, when voices rise or emotions get sharp, a few conscious breaths can keep reactions in check and help you respond rather than react.

The real magic comes when breathwork and body awareness become second nature—a reliable reset button for both frazzled nerves and muddled thoughts. Play with these techniques in different moments, like a busy kitchen, on public transit, or sitting in traffic, and notice which ones bring ease or clarity. There's no wrong way to begin. Every intentional breath is a small act of self-care that ripples through both mind and body.

JOURNALING FOR CLARITY, PURPOSE, AND GROWTH

There's something powerful about putting pen to paper, or even thumb to phone screen, that goes far beyond venting about your day. Journaling, in its many forms, bridges the gap between your thoughts and your body in a way few other habits can. When you write about what's swirling in your head, you're not just organizing words. You're helping your nervous system sort through chaos, soften anxiety, and even calm your racing heart. Science backs this up. Expressive writing has been shown to lower stress, improve sleep, and, in some studies, even boost immune response. One research review found that people who journaled about their emotions experienced improvements in both physical symptoms and overall well-being compared to those who didn't (Reid 2024).

It's not just theory. Real people see these effects every day. We'll never forget one reader who shared her experience with us. She'd been side-lined by a major health setback, her body didn't move the way it used to, and frustration boiled over. At first, she scribbled angry, messy notes in a cheap notebook just to get it all out. This led to longer periods of writing where she described more about her frustrations and suffering. Over time, she noticed something unexpected. Her sleep improved on nights she journaled, and her blood pressure was lower at her next checkup. She started using her journal as both a safe space for tough emotions and a logbook for little victories, like "I walked to the mailbox today without pain." Small shifts like these added up, helping her rebuild confidence and see herself as resilient, not broken.

The beauty of journaling is that you don't need to be a writer or stick to "dear diary" entries. Mix it up with prompts that go deeper than recapping your day. Try asking yourself: "What signals is my body giving me today?" Maybe you notice tension in your shoulders or butterflies in your stomach, jot it down. Another favorite is "What emotion is most present right now, and where do I feel it physically?" This helps connect feelings with their physical roots so you can spot patterns over time. Or reflect on the meaning: "How did my choices today reflect my values?" Maybe you choose rest over hustle or kindness over criticism. Those tiny choices shape your Wellness Blueprint.

Journaling isn't only for reflection. It's a practical tool for behavior change. Tracking triggers can make invisible habits visible and therefore changeable. Use a trigger log to note when cravings, tension, or fatigue arise during your day. Write down what was happening, who you were with, how you felt in your body, and what you did next. Soon enough, patterns emerge, maybe stress eating always follows tough meetings, or fatigue hits after certain foods. When you spot these trends, you can plan new responses instead of falling into old ruts.

Rigid rules kill the joy of journaling, so ditch the idea that you have to fill pages every day or write in perfect sentences. Micro-journaling makes this habit sustainable for real life. Try jotting down three bullet points at night before bed or voice memos on your phone while walking the dog. Draw doodles if words aren't coming, or use color to capture mood if that's more your style. There's no wrong way to document your inner life. What matters is showing up for yourself in whatever format feels easy, honest, and doable.

Reflection Prompts Menu

- How does my body feel right now? Are there any areas of tension or ease? What might those sensations be trying to tell me?

- When do I feel most connected to my body? What activities or environments help foster that connection?
- What physical symptoms do I notice when I'm stressed, anxious, or overwhelmed? How do I usually respond to them?
- What three ways have I supported my mental and physical well-being this week?
- How do my emotions influence the way I treat my body? How does the state of my body influence my mood or thoughts?
- What does wellness mean to me personally, not by societal standards, but what feels aligned with my life and values?
- Write about a time I felt calm, grounded, and present. What contributed to that state? How can I recreate it more often?
- What beliefs do I hold about my body? Are these beliefs kind, neutral, or critical? Where did they come from?
- How do I nourish myself physically, emotionally, and spiritually? What might need more attention?
- What small, loving action can I take today to support both my mind and body?

Use these prompts when you feel stuck or want to spark insight. Copy them into your notebook or notes app so they're handy when needed.

As this chapter draws to a close, think of journaling as another tool in your wellness kit, a way to check in with yourself, process what matters, and nudge both mind and body toward healing and growth. Though you might not be in touch with your mind-body connection just yet, with consistent practice of the techniques we have seen in this chapter, it won't be long before you can harness the potency of this connection for your wellness. As we move forward, remember that clarity leads to action, setting the stage for building connection and community in wellness, which is where we're headed next.

13

CONNECTION, COMMUNITY, AND BUILDING A SUPPORTIVE ECOSYSTEM

I magine you're sitting in your kitchen, scrolling through your phone, and you suddenly realize you haven't had a real conversation—one of those honest, comfortable talks—in days, maybe even weeks. You wave to neighbors, maybe nod to coworkers in meetings, but something feels off. You crave more than just casual hellos or emoji replies. Maybe it's a little loneliness peeking through, or maybe it's just the itch for something deeper. This is where the social side of wellness comes alive.

THE SOCIAL WELLNESS PILLAR: WHY CONNECTION FUELS HEALTH

Social connection is hardwired into human health. Scientists have found that people with even a few strong relationships live longer, recover faster from stress, and enjoy better moods day to day. A report from the World Health Organization explained how loneliness can increase the risk of stroke, heart disease, diabetes, and double the likelihood of depression. In fact, it's estimated that there are 100 deaths an hour linked to loneliness (World Health Organization 2025). Another study from Stanford's Center for Compassion and Altruism Research and Education shows that people with consistent, supportive relationships have less chronic illness, less depression, and even better immune response (Seppala 2014). When you think about it, being connected is as vital as eating well or moving your body.

You don't need a giant tribe to get these benefits. The magic is in the quality, not the quantity. It's tempting to believe that more friends or followers equals more support, but what truly matters is depth. You might know dozens of people from work, the gym, or your neighborhood, but one close friend who gets you can offer more comfort than a room full of friendly faces. We once heard from a reader, Jen, who lost touch with most of her old friends after moving for a new job. At first, she felt isolated in a new city until she reconnected with an old college buddy over video calls. That one relationship became her lifeline through tough workdays and changes at home. It wasn't the numbers on her contact list that helped. It was knowing someone truly saw her.

This connection isn't just about having someone to vent to. It can fuel your motivation and make healthy habits stick. Another reader, Marcus, wasn't much for gyms or solo jogging. But after joining a local walking group, which had just three people at first, he found himself showing up even on rainy mornings. The group swapped recipes, cheered each other on, and celebrated every little win. Marcus told us that what kept him going wasn't guilt or pressure but the simple joy of knowing someone was waiting for him at the park bench. That's the power of shared commitment.

Interestingly, support is not a one-way street. Both giving and receiving help boost your well-being in unique ways. When you show up for someone else, maybe by checking in on a friend or volunteering at a community garden, your sense of meaning and belonging gets a major lift. Psychologists call it the "helper's high." Brain scans reveal that even thinking about donating money to a charity can increase the area of the brain associated with pleasure (Realized Worth 2021). There's a reader named Priya who started volunteering at her neighborhood garden during a tough year. Pulling weeds together turned into sharing coffee and stories. She left every Saturday feeling lighter and more hopeful than she had all week. Over time, those fellow volunteers became friends she could rely on, and she realized that helping out helped her as much as anyone.

Of course, building or rebuilding connections isn't always easy. Loneliness hits hard, especially after big life changes like moving, changing jobs, or even just growing apart from friends over time. And let's be honest, past hurts can leave scars that make trust tricky. If you're feeling stuck or unsure how to reconnect after drifting apart, it often helps to start small, perhaps a text that says, "Hey, it's been a while. I've been thinking about you and would love to catch up if you're up for it." If you're nervous about the silence between you and an old friend, try something like, "I know it's been ages since we talked, but I miss those conversations we used to have." Many people feel relieved by honesty and happy to reconnect, even if it takes a little time to rebuild that rhythm.

Social anxiety can make reaching out feel risky. Social anxiety is a persistent fear of being judged, embarrassed, or negatively evaluated in social situations. It can make everyday interactions, like starting a conversation or speaking in a group, feel overwhelming. One evidence-based way to manage social anxiety is gradual exposure, where individuals slowly and intentionally face the situations they fear in a controlled, step-by-step way. For example, someone who feels anxious about speaking in public might start by practicing a short speech alone, then progress to presenting in front of a mirror, then to a close friend, and eventually to a small group. Each step builds confidence and reduces fear by showing the brain that the situation is not as threatening as it once seemed. Over time, this repeated exposure can help rewire the brain's response to social triggers, making social situations feel less intimidating and more manageable (Smith 2023).

Reflection Exercise: Mapping Your Connection Needs

Grab your journal and write down three relationships where you feel truly seen or supported, even if they're not frequent contacts right now. What makes those connections special? Next, jot down one person you'd like to reconnect with or get to know better. What's one simple way you could reach out this week, either by text, call, or a coffee invite? Finally, reflect on ways you already give support (maybe helping a neighbor or listening to a friend vent) and how those moments make you feel.

Social wellness isn't about popularity contests. It's about genuine belonging and shared care. Whether your circle is wide or close-knit, whether you reach out first or accept help when it's offered, connection is a powerful force shaping your health and your happiness right now.

FINDING YOUR WELLNESS TRIBE: SUPPORT, ACCOUNTABILITY, AND BELONGING

Finding your wellness tribe goes beyond having a few gym buddies or an occasional group chat. It's about connecting with people who genuinely understand your goals and want to see you succeed. A wellness tribe offers an invisible safety net. You don't have to justify your healthy choices like walking more, cooking at home, or skipping late-night take-out. Shared goals and values bind you together, keeping you motivated when things get tough.

A wellness tribe could be as small as two or three people who truly care about each other's progress. These are the friends who ask how you're doing and mean it, who offer encouragement when you skip a workout, and celebrate every win, big or small. The magic is in shared values, even if your exact routines differ. Maybe you all want to move more, eat better, manage stress, or simply build steadier habits. The main thing is that you're in it together.

IDENTIFYING SHARED INTERESTS OR WELLNESS GOALS

Go back to your journal and the lists of what excites you or areas you want to improve. Consider friends, coworkers, or neighbors who talk about these interests. Perhaps it's the colleague who heads out for a lunchtime walk, someone who brings healthy lunches, or the friendly dog park regular. If you can't think of anyone, don't worry, your future tribe could still be out there.

Building new connections can be intimidating, especially if you've been alone or had negative group experiences in the past. Luckily, there are many ways to find your people. Local options, often overlooked, can be very welcoming. Yoga studios usually have beginner classes with zero expectation for perfection. Group fitness classes offer natural account-ability as you see the same faces week after week, making it easier to strike up conversations. Book clubs that focus on health or personal growth attract people seeking more than just small talk. Running and walking groups (even the walk/run ones) are great for connecting.

Online communities provide even more options. Wellness forums allow you to ask questions and share wins without worrying about appear-ances. Social media groups can be great sources of encouragement and advice. Virtual challenges, like step counts tracked together via apps or meal prep streaks, unite people from everywhere. Start small by commenting on posts or introducing yourself in a thread—sometimes that's enough to begin a real connection.

If you want to bring someone into your wellness world, start with someone you trust, a friend, sibling, coworker, or even an online acquaintance. Look for qualities that matter: supportive, nonjudgmen-tal, reliable, and open about their own ups and downs. Avoid anyone who shames mistakes or turns every check-in into a lecture. When you're ready, keep it simple. Try something like, "Hey, would you like to check in weekly about our wellness wins? Nothing fancy, just support and encouragement." Or, "I'm trying to walk more and could use a buddy to share progress with. Interested?" If you need a checklist for picking the right partner, look for:

- Trustworthiness and a sense of responsibility.
- Willingness to celebrate effort (not just outcomes).
- Flexibility about plans and schedules.
- Ability to listen without fixing.
- A sense of humor for those inevitable off days.

Once you've found your person (or small group), talk through how you'll connect. Weekly check-ins work well for many, whether it's a quick call, text thread, or voice memo swap. Decide if you'd like daily nudges ("Did you move today?"), more reflective sharing ("What felt good/what flopped?"), or just "Yay!" messages for wins. You could use shared digital logs or group chats, where each person posts daily victories, think of it as a rolling celebration board. For those who like structure, set a recurring wellness wins call every Sunday night or agree on monthly coffee dates (in person or virtual) to toast progress. Even quick video calls can spark joy and keep goals fresh. The real work comes after you've found your tribe. Remember that maintaining these relationships takes effort, but it shouldn't feel like another chore.

Trust deepens over time, not from grand gestures, but by showing up consistently and being open about both setbacks and successes. Don't be afraid to admit when you're struggling. Letting others see your real ups and downs encourages them to do the same. These moments gradually build genuine loyalty and support, both for wellness goals and for other life challenges.

Stories from readers highlight the power of this belonging. One reached a plateau after endless solo workouts and meal planning. Everything shifted after joining a workplace step challenge, where coworkers encouraged each other not just with steps, but with memes, playlists, and snack ideas. She broke her plateau and rediscovered joy in her workplace thanks to the camaraderie.

Another parent felt isolated in her meal prep until joining an online group focused on family-friendly batch cooking. Trading dinner photos (successes and flops) helped her gain tips, support, and real friendship beyond recipes. She told us that she credits the group for helping her stick with her goals and stay sane during chaos.

Your wellness tribe doesn't need to look a certain way. It just needs to feel right. Whether in person or online, big or small, formal or casual, the belonging and support will propel you farther than willpower alone ever could.

BOUNDARIES AND BALANCE TO PROTECT YOUR ENERGY IN RELATIONSHIPS

Boundaries aren't there to shut others out but to safeguard your energy from being depleted by overcommitment or others' demands. Instead of seeing them as cold, imagine them as barriers to preserve your ability to grow, thrive, and share what's healthy inside. Without them, you risk feeling drained, resentful from saying yes too often, or burned out from putting yourself last. If family weekends exhaust you or a friend's constant messages annoy you, your boundaries may need reinforcing.

Honoring your limits is self-respect in action and essential for sustainable wellness. When you constantly give away your energy, you're left with little for self-care or joy. You may even notice that you struggle to meet your basic needs, like sleep and eating well. This emptiness breeds resentment, making generosity and love harder to give. Boundaries prevent this slow drain. They gently signal, "This is what I need to stay healthy and happy." Sometimes, it's taking thirty minutes alone after work before socializing. Other times, it's declining a last-minute plan to protect your sleep or workout routine. Here are the main types of boundaries and how they relate to wellness.

- **Mental Boundaries:** Protect your thoughts, values, and opinions.
  - Saying "I respect your view, but I disagree" during a wellness discussion.
  - Choosing not to engage in negative self-talk or diet culture conversations.
- **Emotional Boundaries:** Protect your feelings and emotional well-being.
  - Telling a friend, "I'm not in the right headspace to talk about that right now."
  - Refusing to take responsibility for someone else's emotional state.
- **Physical Boundaries:** Protect your personal space and physical needs.
  - Declining a hug when you're not comfortable with it.
  - Prioritizing sleep or rest over attending a late-night event.
- **Time Boundaries:** Protect how you spend your time.
  - Setting specific "me time" for exercise or meditation.
  - Blocking out thirty minutes daily for meal prep or mindful eating.

- **Digital Boundaries:** Protect your online engagement and screen time.
  - Turning off notifications after a certain hour to protect your mental space.
  - Unfollowing accounts that promote unhealthy body standards.
- **Material Boundaries:** Protect your money and possessions.
  - Saying no to lending your wellness gear (e.g., yoga mat) if you're not comfortable.
  - Creating a budget for wellness activities that aligns with your priorities (Center for Mindful Psychotherapy 2023).

Start identifying your boundaries with honest reflection. Notice what leaves you tired or tense and what interactions or routines make you feel recharged. Write down your answers to the following prompts to help you, as these are the places where your boundaries need to be strengthened.

- When do I feel most drained or overwhelmed? What boundary might have been crossed?
- What situations or people make me feel uncomfortable or anxious? Why?
- Do I ever say "yes" when I really want to say "no"? What stops me?
- What do I need more of in my daily life to feel balanced and well?
- How do I react when someone disagrees with me or pushes my limits?
- How do I protect my emotional energy in relationships?
- Are there relationships in my life that consistently leave me feeling guilty, anxious, or exhausted?
- How do I prioritize my own wellness needs, even when others make demands on my time?
- What parts of my routine are nonnegotiable for my health (sleep, meals, movement, quiet time)?

- When was the last time I did something just for me? How can I do that more often?

Expressing boundaries takes practice, but it's easier with clear language and self-compassion. Use simple scripts if you feel unsure: "I want to be present with you, but I need thirty minutes to myself first," or "I'm not able to help this week. I need time to recharge." Remember, no one else can guard your energy for you. Notice how each of these phrases starts with "I." These "I" statements are essential for communicating healthy boundaries. They keep the focus on your needs and hold you account-able for your emotions (Vossenkemper, n.d.). Imagine how someone would take "You are overwhelming me and I need an afternoon to myself," compared with "I am feeling overwhelmed and I need an after-noon to myself." It's a subtle difference, but enough to prevent someone from becoming defensive.

Setting boundaries can trigger resistance, especially when people are used to your constant yes. Friends might act surprised or disappointed, family may guilt you, or vice versa. This is normal. The urge to please everyone is strong, especially if you were taught that self-sacrifice is admirable. But you're not selfish for needing space. You're wise for protecting your well-being. Stick to calm, consistent statements: "I can't make it tonight, but I hope you all have fun." Avoid apologizing because your well-being isn't something to feel guilty about. If people continue to cross your boundaries, it's worth considering the consequences and sticking to them, or else these people will never learn to respect your limits.

During busy periods like holidays or work deadlines, boundaries matter even more. You may face increased demands, from family events to extra projects at work. Respond simply and firmly with phrases like "I can't add more right now." For family pressure, try, "I'll join after my walk," or "I'll leave at eight to rest." Stay consistent, and most people will adapt once they see your boundaries are real.

Boundaries need regular attention as they're not a one-time task. As life changes, your needs change too. Regular boundary audits help. Each month, ask yourself where you felt stretched too thin or disrespected, and what you'd like to change. While it's possible you may need to set new boundaries, you may also find that some of your existing boundaries can be relaxed.

Major life transitions often test boundaries: a new boss who messages outside work hours, the demands of new parenthood, or living with a partner who unintentionally overwhelms your calendar. These moments call for recalibration. Adjust your limits as needed. If you slip up and let a boundary slide, don't dwell on guilt. Instead, use it as information for next time. What made you say yes, and what would help you say no?

Clear limits and honest talk let you show up fully for others and for yourself. Protecting your space supports every wellness area. Sleep, movement, nutrition, and connection all thrive with good boundaries. As we continue, we'll see how nature, purpose, and joy bring wholeness, showing that wellness is about more than just getting by. It's about feeling truly alive.

14

NATURE, PURPOSE, AND JOY BEYOND THE BASICS

I magine you're in the middle of a packed week, your mind buzzing with tasks and your shoulders tight from too many hours indoors. You glance out a window and catch a glimpse of a tree swaying or a patch of blue sky. For a moment, you feel your breath deepen. There's a reason this tiny pause feels like a relief. You don't need to hike a mountain or venture into deep forests to reap nature's benefits. Even a sliver of sunlight or a single pot of herbs by your sink can make a difference.

NATURE AS MEDICINE: INCORPORATING THE OUTDOORS FOR MIND AND BODY

Research increasingly validates the benefits of nature on mental health. Spending time in green spaces, from forests to parks, has been shown to improve creativity, focus, and attention, alleviate symptoms of anxiety and depression, and boost heart health. Time outdoors doesn't just help the mind—it supports your immune system too. Sunlight hitting your skin helps produce vitamin D, which supports bone health and immune response (UCLA Health 2025).

The practice of forest bathing, originating from the Japanese shinrin-yoku, underscores these benefits by demonstrating how immersion in forest environments reduces stress-related cortisol levels, leading to a natural relaxation of the body's stress responses. This was backed in a systematic review of twenty-two articles, all confirming that cortisol levels were significantly lower after forest bathing (Association of Nature and Forest Therapy, n.d.). It's not about hiking or exercising but rather about mindfully connecting with nature through all your senses. To practice forest bathing, find a quiet, wooded area and walk slowly and calmly without any specific destination. Focus on the sights, sounds, smells, and textures around you, like the rustling of leaves, the scent of pine, or the feeling of moss under your fingers. You can find a spot to sit for a while and practice deep breathing or other relaxation techniques. Leave distractions behind (for safety reasons, take your phone but switch it off), and allow yourself to simply be present.

But maybe you're thinking, "That sounds great for people with hiking trails nearby, but I live in an apartment," or "My mobility isn't what it used to be." The good news is you can connect with nature anywhere. If you're in an apartment, try balcony gardening. A few pots of basil or hardy succulents are enough to bring green to your day. No balcony? Place plants near your window so you can see them while working or relaxing. Indoor plants are shown to boost mood and purify air (The Sill, n.d.). If gardening isn't your thing, simply gazing out the window at the sky, trees, or even passing clouds offers a micro-dose of calm. Studies have highlighted how even looking at images of nature can increase parasympathetic activity and calm your nervous system (Brown et al. 2013).

Suburban life brings its own opportunities. Take lunch breaks to the nearest patch of grass. An urban park, community garden, or even a quiet median strip with flowers can give you a break from concrete and car horns. If walking isn't easy for you, sit on a bench or lay a blanket out and let yourself soak up the sights and sounds. For those with limited mobility or who spend much of the day inside, nature gazing is powerful. Sit by a window, notice the shifting light, watch birds flutter by, or let your attention rest on the shapes of leaves. It sounds simple, but these moments retrain the mind to slow down.

Any chance you have, take your shoes off and place your bare feet on the ground, like forest bathing. This may at first seem a little hippie, but it's another science-backed strategy for your wellness. Earthing, also known as grounding, is the practice of physically connecting your body to the earth's natural surface, typically by walking barefoot on grass, soil, sand, or even immersing yourself in water. Again, if mobility is an issue, you can still soak up the earth's natural energy by sitting down and connecting to the ground, or you could use indoor earthing mats. The concept is based on the idea that the earth's surface carries a subtle electrical charge, and by making direct contact with it, we can absorb electrons that may help neutralize free radicals and reduce inflammation in the body. Emerging research suggests that earthing may offer several health benefits, including improved sleep, reduced stress levels, better mood, and it could counteract cardiovascular, neurodegenerative, respiratory, and autoimmune conditions (Fischer 2024). Whether it's a barefoot walk in a park, gardening with your hands in the soil, or lying on the beach, incorporating regular moments of earthing into your wellness routine can support both physical and emotional balance.

If you want to make nature part of your everyday rhythm, try building outdoor rituals. Routines help us stick with what makes us feel good, even when we're busy. Maybe you drink your morning coffee on the porch or steps instead of at the kitchen table. This tiny shift makes waking up feel fresh and intentional. Try using a sunset signal. When the sky changes color at day's end, pause work and step outside for a few breaths, marking the transition from hustle to rest. You could commit to a weekly outdoor activity challenge. One week, it could be laying out for a picnic lunch (even if it's just a sandwich on a towel in the backyard); another week, it's trying out birdwatching (no fancy tools needed, just curiosity), or simply finding a new walking route.

Interactive Element: Nature Reflection Exercise

Next time you are outside or near an open window, jot down what you notice in a nature journal entry. What scents drift by? How does the air feel on your skin? Did anything surprise you, like a sudden breeze, a butterfly landing nearby? If you're able, slip off your shoes and stand barefoot on grass or sand for two minutes for an unexpected sense of peace.

Nature's medicine is available to all of us, from sunlight through glass to the smell of rain on pavement. When you intentionally invite these moments into your routine and tune your attention to them, you'll likely uncover new reserves of calm and clarity within yourself.

ALIGNING WELLNESS WITH PURPOSE AND VALUES-BASED LIVING

Waking up with a sense of direction is vitalizing. Don't think this means having your entire life planned out. It's about knowing what really matters to you. Purpose isn't just a motivational cliché. Instead, it shapes how you feel, move through the world, and handle stress. Science repeatedly shows that people with a clear sense of purpose live longer, recover faster, and stay motivated, especially when life gets hard. There is now evidence that links a sense of purpose to a longer life (Berman 2022). In Blue Zones, where residents often live into their nineties, a key thread is an active sense of meaning, often described by the Japanese word "ikigai," a combination of "iki" (meaning life) and "gai" (meaning worth or purpose). It's a traditional belief that physical wellness is impacted by mental wellness and a sense of purpose in life (Gaines 2020).

Purpose transcends grand missions and can manifest in the simplicity of being a reliable parent or the depth of artistic creation and altruism. Your sense of purpose requires you to align daily actions with your core interests. Values, like honesty, creativity, and kindness, guide this alignment like an internal compass. To identify your values, envision a deck of cards, each representing a value such as family, growth, or humor. Select the five you deem indispensable. Alternatively, consider, "What do I want my legacy to be?" Let your thoughts flow freely, listing ideals like generosity or the impact of raising resilient children. There are no incorrect responses, and gaining clarity may require time.

Once you know your core values, let them guide your decisions, especially during daily challenges. You begin to see which habits align with your values and which don't. For example, if connection matters to you but your calendar's full of draining social events, you'll likely feel exhausted and resentful. If you value presence but are always tired from late nights, it may be time to skip late-night unhealthy habits and prioritize sleep so you're actually present for family conversations. Values help you distinguish between genuine self-care and trendy should-dos. Ask yourself, "Does this fit what matters most to me?" If not, it's okay to let it go.

This act of wellness can be enhanced when combined with habit stacking with intention and using your values as the filter, not adding random new behaviors. For example, before starting a new workout or diet, check if it matches your core values. Maybe movement's best for you when done with friends (community), or when it lets you reflect (growth). No need to overhaul your life overnight. Even one small values-based tweak deepens your sense of purpose.

As you align your life with your values, motivation shifts from being an uphill battle to feeling like a gentle pull in the right direction. There will always be setbacks and imperfect days. But when your choices reflect what matters most to you, small wins are satisfying and setbacks hurt less because you're still heading true north.

Reflection Prompt: Values-to-Action Roadmap

Take five minutes to write down two of your top values. For each, brainstorm one small action you could take this week to reflect that value in your wellness routine. For instance, if generosity is important, share a home-cooked meal or offer a walk for a neighbor who needs support. If adventure excites you, try a new walking route or a beginner's dance class just for fun. Wellness is about living on purpose, not just checking boxes.

INFUSING JOY AND PLAY: THE SECRET INGREDIENTS OF SUSTAINABLE HEALTH

Somewhere along the way, many of us picked up the idea that adulthood is all about getting things done, checking off lists, and being serious most of the time. Laughter and play end up squeezed into the margins, if they happen at all. But here's something you might not hear enough. Fun is not a luxury. It's not just for kids or reserved for vacations. Joy and playfulness are immense tools for your health, more so if you want wellness to last. Science backs this up, too. Studies on laughter therapy show that frequent laughter can lower blood pressure, boost heart health, increase heart rate, and improve blood flow, reducing the risk of stroke and heart disease. When you laugh, your body releases serotonin and dopamine, those all-important feel-good chemicals. A good laugh can also improve sleep and potentially help with pain management (Better Help 2025). Play isn't just a break from stress. It can be an antidote.

Despite the numerous benefits, many adults struggle to engage in fun activities without feeling guilty or self-conscious, hindered by the misconception that play is frivolous or a waste of time. Concerns about appearing silly or facing judgment, coupled with the relentless demands of work and family responsibilities, often relegate leisure to the bottom of the priority list.

So, how do you give yourself permission to play? Affirmations can play an important role. Try repeating, "Today I'm allowed to have fun, no guilt, no apology." Say it aloud, stick it on your fridge, or keep it in your wallet. If your brain tries to talk you out of joy with old stories about productivity or embarrassment, remember that joy is fuel, not fluff.

There is no single right way to have fun and laugh. Play is personal. If you're extroverted, maybe you get a kick out of hosting game nights or organizing a dance party with friends or family. Put on music (even if it's cheesy), let the kids or roommates join in, and see who has the goofiest moves. If you're more introverted or need solo time, try puzzles, painting, singing in the shower, or building something with your hands. Creative hobbies count as play, too. Consider sketching cartoons, decorating cookies, building models, or picking up an instrument you haven't touched in years. We all keep a folder on our phones, and any meme or video we share that makes us laugh goes into our folder. This is a great way to keep things personal, appreciating that not everyone's humor is the same. Any time one of us needs a quick laugh, we can pop into our own folders.

The real trick is not to overthink it. Play doesn't need to be scheduled or perfect. Even five minutes of spontaneous silliness counts. Try setting aside a little time each week for something that's just for fun where the only goal is to enjoy yourself.

If this all feels strange at first, that's perfectly normal. You may have spent years putting your playful side on mute. But every small act of joy is like a snowball effect where the last rolls into the next.

When you build more laughter and lightness into your days, health becomes less about discipline and more about delight. Motivation sticks around longer when it's tied to pleasure instead of duty. Now that we've explored how nature, purpose, and joy shape real wellness, we'll shift our focus to bringing these lessons into everyday routines, making wellness more lasting in the context of daily life.

15

THE WELLNESS BLUEPRINT IN ACTION

Change for Life

Not so long ago, the world was minding its own business when, all of a sudden, chaos struck, and few could escape it. Panic buying led to food shortages, gyms shut down, and many were confined to their homes. The pandemic is the perfect example of how we can be going about our daily lives, and, through no fault of our own, wellness gets put on the back burner. Remember the challenges you faced during the pandemic? It wasn't easy to stick to the usual routine, was it? You never know what is around the corner, which means you need a plan that's ready for any surprise the future holds.

YOUR PERSONALIZED WELLNESS ROADMAP: BUILDING AND UPDATING YOUR PLAN

Start by drawing your own wellness roadmap. Treat it like a mind map with five sections: nutrition, movement, sleep, mindset, and connection. Under each, jot down what truly works for you, not what's trendy or expected. Maybe nutrition means batch cooking soup on Sundays instead of perfect meal prep. For movement, perhaps a twenty-minute walk after lunch is better than gym sessions. Be honest about sleep. Would moving your phone out of the room help? For mindset, a simple sentence of gratitude before bed might be enough. Connection can be as easy as texting a cousin once a week, not going to large gatherings.

After building your roadmap, check in with it regularly. Every few months or after major changes, do a wellness audit. Honestly assess what feels easy, what feels tough, and where you feel stuck. Use prompts like "Where am I thriving effortlessly?" and "What feels forced?" If life shifts, such as starting a new commute, adding responsibilities, or a family member needs more care, commit to adjusting. During these moments of adjustments, it's wise to turn to those batch meals you made in the freezer instead of feeling the pressure of having to cook fresh meals. One reader, after switching jobs, had to give up his evening swims because of a change in schedule. Because of his mindset, he didn't give up on exercise. He chose to go to bed earlier so that he could start waking up earlier and enjoy a morning swim.

Distinguish between micro-goals and big-picture dreams. Micro-goals are small, daily wins like adding more antioxidants to your diet, taking the stairs, and turning off screens ten minutes earlier. Your bigger goals are your north star. They are about how you want to feel and live. Let's look at a practical example. Say your bigger goal is to hike the Grand Canyon Rim-to-Rim trail in two years. You aren't going to reach this goal unless you break it down and start working on your mini-goals, perhaps starting with a three-mile walk and adding a mile every other week. The mini-goal is achievable. There is room for adjustments in case of setbacks, but at the same time, there is also the real possibility of hitting these mini-goals ahead of time.

Interactive Reflection: Planning Your Goals

Complete the following sentences to clarify your goals:

In two years, I want to achieve _____

_____

In order to do this, I need to _____

_____

To achieve my mini-goals, today I will _____

_____

HABIT TRACKERS, CHECKLISTS, AND TEMPLATES: TOOLS FOR EVERYDAY SUCCESS

You know those days when you're not sure if you actually drank enough water or moved more than from your desk to the fridge? That's where tracking tools become your guide and motivation. You don't need to love spreadsheets or journals to get results—there's a tool for every style. Some folks get a kick out of coloring in a twenty-one-day mindful minutes chart, others prefer ticking boxes on a weekly movement log, while tech lovers gravitate toward habit tracker apps that ping reminders and give out badges. Seeing those rows of checkmarks or gold stars has a way of making you want to keep the streak alive.

The joy comes from tailoring these tools to your own quirks and preferences. If you're creative and love color, print a big tracker and use stickers or doodles to mark off habits. If lists calm your mind, a daily checklist with simple boxes to tick as you go can be satisfying. Tech fans might want a digital app that lets you track habits, moods, and even streaks; some sync with your calendar so you don't forget.

Try this as an example of a simple weekly habit tracker.

Habit	Mon	Tue	Wed	Thur	Fri	Sat	Sun	Reward

Be sure to customize your chart for the number of habits you want to track. Just because there are seven rows here, it doesn't mean you need to jump in with seven habits. At the same time, you may want to add more. Notice the final column? Don't forget to set a specific reward so that you can celebrate each win and keep your momentum going.

Consistency is easier when you celebrate even tiny wins. Some people set up a "sticker system"—each day you complete a habit, slap on a sticker. It feels playful, but it's backed by science: Those little rewards are like mini high-fives for your brain. After seven days, take a minute to jot down what felt easy, what tripped you up, and what you want to adjust. Don't be hard on yourself. This is your opportunity to learn and make the necessary tweaks.

Sometimes tracking can feel like just another chore. If you ever find yourself dreading your tracker or losing steam, simplify. Use a bare minimum checklist for weeks when life gets hectic. Focus on one or two habits that matter most and let the rest go for now. There's no rule that says you need to track everything all the time. At the end of each month, refresh your template, maybe change colors, switch from paper to digital (or the other way around), or try a new format completely. Keeping things fresh helps prevent boredom.

OVERCOMING WELLNESS FATIGUE: STAYING INSPIRED YEAR AFTER YEAR

Even the most motivated people hit a wall sometimes. You might notice routines that once energized you now feel dull, or you wake up already tired at the thought of another salad or workout. Maybe you're just going through the motions, checking boxes but not feeling any spark. Wellness fatigue sneaks in quietly. It can show up as restlessness, loss of excitement about progress, even a bit of resentment or dread around habits you used to enjoy. You find yourself sighing at your meal prep, dragging your feet on walks, or skipping check-ins because what's the point? These are warning signs of wellness fatigue.

When that flat feeling settles in, it's time to shake things up. One strategy is a seasonal refresh. Each season brings its own flavors and possibilities. Think spring salads, summer hikes, cozy autumn soups, or winter stretching beside a window. Change up your recipes, experiment with new movement styles, or set a playful mini-challenge. Take advantage of seasonal fruits and vegetables as part of a challenge. Try adding a different fruit or veg in each season. Or you join a group challenge, virtual or in person, for a dose of external energy and friendly accountability.

Don't underestimate the power of rest and play. Sometimes, the best thing you can do is schedule a full break from your wellness goals. Mark a day or weekend on your calendar just for fun, maybe that's painting, exploring a new café, hosting a game night, or whatever feels light and unrelated to wellness checklists. Give yourself real permission to skip routines or pare them down to the bare minimum for a short period. This isn't losing ground. It's fueling up for what's next. If this feels too guilty for you, time your rest after hitting a goal and treat it as your reward.

Other times, you may just need to discover fresh inspiration. Perhaps your affirmations are no longer having the same impact, your mind is bored with the same visualization imagery, or your goals have slipped into things you should be doing instead of what to do. A vision board could provide you with this fresh inspiration. Look for new quotes, images of unknown places, and different scenes, and check out things like recipes and music from other cultures. Take these items you collect and add them to a vision board. Update your vision board as and when you need to remain inspired so your long-term goals stay fresh.

TEACHING AND LEADING: SHARING YOUR BLUEPRINT WITH OTHERS

Every small step toward wellness can have a profound impact, often igniting a ripple effect of health consciousness. For instance, adopting simple habits like packing a nutritious lunch, embracing walks in all weathers, or taking moments for mindfulness can inspire others to follow suit. It's the quiet, consistent actions that often wield the most influence. At our office, one of our colleagues switched to a standing desk. They raved about the potential benefits like better posture, less neck and back pain, and more focus (Kiley 2025). We started to notice they were more active, walking around while on the phone, and they were happier at work. One more standing desk popped up, then another, and we were all in a better mood.

When you want to encourage healthy habits in others, empathy and curiosity get you further than lectures ever will. Instead of telling someone what they should do, invite them in. "Would you like to join me for a Sunday mindful walk?" is much more welcoming than "You should be more mindful." Share your favorite tools, like a meal prep hack or a fitness app, not as prescriptions but as stories. Let them know how the tool has made your life easier, perhaps offering a tip on how to use it. Keep the vibe open-ended and judgment-free.

It's easy to slip into fix-it mode when you're excited about your progress, but it's important to respect where others are in their own process. Sometimes that means holding back on advice unless asked. You might say, "Here's what's working for me right now," rather than implying your way is the only way. If a friend vents about being tired but isn't ready to change, listen without jumping in to solve it. Focus on sharing your experience rather than directing theirs. Your role is to model self-care, not carry the weight of their choices.

If you're looking for ways to spread wellness in your circle, start small and keep it fun. Set up a Wellness Wins Jar in the kitchen or the office so that everyone can drop in slips of paper celebrating something positive they did for their health that week. Try a neighborhood gardening club. No pressure, just show up and perhaps share some seeds or even fresh produce you have grown each week. Or launch a virtual book club focused on self-improvement reads. Pick titles that spark conversations about habits, resilience, or finding joy in ordinary days. When everyone gets to chime in with their successes and struggles, it builds support.

The truth is, teaching and leading in wellness doesn't mean you have to know all the answers. It's about being real, sharing what lights you up, and making space for others to join you on their own terms. Small acts, an invitation here, a story there, can plant seeds that grow into something bigger than you expected.

THE WELLNESS MOVEMENT: IGNITING CHANGE IN YOUR COMMUNITY

You might be surprised how quickly a single idea can ripple outward, reshaping the vibe in your neighborhood, workplace, or even your kid's school. Take, for example, a teacher we know who started weaving short mindfulness breaks into her classroom, just three minutes of quiet breathing after recess. Students went from bouncing off the walls to settling in, and soon other teachers followed suit. Or picture a reader who convinced a handful of neighbors to help clean up a local park. They added a group yoga stretch afterward, drawing in more folks each time. That patch of green went from neglected to cherished, all because someone dared to send a group text and bring a yoga mat.

Organizing community wellness activities need not be daunting. Begin with small initiatives, such as a monthly wellness walk on a safe, accessible route, ensuring it's inclusive for all, including those with strollers and wheelchairs. For workplaces, consider a wellness day featuring healthy snacks, a talk by a local health expert, and simple group activities like stretching or laughter yoga. To streamline planning, create a checklist covering essentials like permissions, refreshments, entertainment, and a weather contingency plan. Be prepared for potential challenges like low attendance or inclement weather. Embrace these as learning opportunities, adapt, and persist with a positive spirit.

As you think bigger, keep inclusion at the heart of your plans. Wellness isn't just for the privileged or the able-bodied. The pandemic highlighted racial discrimination on a global level, and that's only one minority group (Mheidly et al. 2022). We can each make it our social responsibility to welcome all backgrounds and abilities into our wellness plans. When planning an event, ask yourself if people of different ages and cultures can participate. Are there ramps for wheelchairs? What about single parents? You might want to consider a policy that encourages inclusive language. Can you partner with local organizations that reach folks who might not come otherwise? If you're asking for contributions or supplies, make sure there are no hidden costs that could keep people away.

How you spread the word doesn't have to be challenging. Community boards are a great place to reach out to locals. Social media gives you platforms to reach a larger audience, as well as the locals. These sites are also an ideal place for sharing success stories and offering each other further support. Encourage others to share events too. Collective action multiplies impact. Everyone's tiny efforts add up to lasting change.

As this chapter wraps up, remember that sparking wellness in your community doesn't require perfection or big budgets. It just takes one person to start, and you can be that person. These little sparks build the kind of supportive culture where everyone can thrive.

YOUR OPINION MATTERS DEEPLY TO US!

The great thing about reviews is that we get to hear your thoughts and experiences, but they do more than this. People want to hear from others who know what they are talking about, someone they can relate to...and that is you! You might not think your words can make that much of a difference, but for someone who is battling health issues, they can be the light at the end of the tunnel.

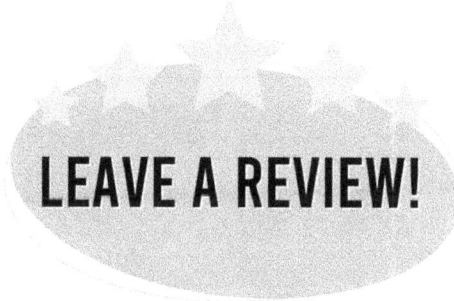

LEAVE A REVIEW!

We are so grateful for the brief time you take out of your day to help. Keep up all your good efforts, be kind to yourself, and remember that your wellness is a priority, not a luxury!

Scan the QR code below

CONCLUSION

You have done something remarkable. You've shown up for yourself. You've carved out time, brought curiosity, and stuck with your individual wellness plan, even on days when your to-do list was screaming louder than your wellness goals. Seriously, take a second and let that soak in. Progress isn't always loud or flashy. Sometimes, it's just quietly turning the page, absorbing information.

Let's circle back to the vision that's been the heartbeat of this book. Wellness isn't a frantic reaction to a crisis. It's not about chasing trends, punishing yourself, or trying to fit into someone else's mold. It's about giving yourself permission to build health from the inside out, one thoughtful choice at a time. It's about becoming the architect of your own vitality, crafting a blueprint that fits your life, your values, your wild schedule, and your unique hopes. You have that agency. You always have, even if the world sometimes tries to convince you otherwise.

Throughout these chapters, we've explored the big pillars that shape real, lasting wellness. We started with your mindset, because how you talk to yourself matters. It's the difference between a supportive coach and a relentless critic. We dug into habit science, learning that tiny steps and micro-goals beat grand plans that fizzle within months, if not weeks.

We reimagined nutrition, not as a restrictive chore, but as flexible, joyful fuel. For too long, we have been influenced by fad diets that may work for the few but don't take into account the individual needs of the human body. Movement became about daily life, not just gym sessions. It's amazing how even our daily chores can be turned into moderate physical activity when you turn on the tunes and increase the intensity of your moves. The cycle became complete when we covered the need for quality sleep. You might not notice it on day one, but it won't be long before your diet gives you more energy to work out and, in turn, you get to sleep better and wake up feeling refreshed.

We tackled stress with practical tools for resilience like tiny pauses, mindful breathing, and self-compassion scripts. All of this was helped with a dash of science, just enough to understand how the body responds to stress and how to stimulate your vagus nerve to increase parasympathetic activity. It's the vagus nerve that helps us appreciate the mind-body connection. Don't forget to feed your second brain with probiotics and prebiotics for a holistic approach to your wellness plan.

We didn't stop there. We looked at digital wellness and the importance of setting healthy boundaries with our screens, instead of letting them steal our rest or joy. We talked about progress tracking, not for perfection's sake, but to celebrate the wins that often go unseen. We celebrated the power of community—how connection, support, and shared accountability turn solo goals into lasting change. And we stepped outside the basics, embracing nature, purpose, and joy as vital nutrients for your soul. All of this, stitched together, is what makes wellness real, sustainable, and—let's be honest—way more fun.

Personalization was our north star. Your wellness plan should flex, shift, and grow as you do. And we faced setbacks head-on, learning to recalibrate (not restart), and starting fresh with mini-goals are all part of your progress, and nothing to feel ashamed or guilty about.

So what are the big takeaways? First, progress always wins over perfection. You don't have to get it right every day. What matters is showing up, adapting, and being kind to yourself when life throws curveballs. Second, self-compassion isn't fluff; it's fuel. Talking to yourself like you'd talk to a good friend changes everything. Third, celebrating your wins, big and small, is a must. It fills you with a sense of pride and keeps you motivated. On the days that you feel like you have failed, remember you haven't, because tomorrow is a new day.

Maybe you've tried new routines, reflected on old habits, or even scribbled a few wins into a jar. Maybe you've just started noticing your own patterns with a little more kindness. That's real progress. That's how change happens—one choice, one reflection, one honest moment at a time.

Here's what we're inviting you to do next. Take the blueprint you've been building and put it into your real, messy, beautiful life. Use the trackers, checklists, and reflection questions. Don't wait for a perfect Monday. Start where you are, with what you have. Keep what works, tweak what doesn't, and don't be afraid to start small.

And please, don't go it alone. Find an accountability buddy, join a wellness tribe, or invite your family or colleagues to try one small change together. Share your wins, your struggles, and your favorite hacks. The more we lift each other up, the easier it gets for everyone. Wellness is contagious, in the best way.

Speaking of lifting each other up, we have a small ask of you. Considering the prevalence of chronic conditions, the lack of diversity in the global healthcare system, and the fact that some people have such limited resources, there is a way you can help. One honest opinion of this book on Amazon can enable other people who are struggling with their wellness to see that there are practical and effective strategies. It's another way that we can add to the community of wellness, share stories, and celebrate together.

You've got a powerful voice. Use it to make wellness accessible and inclusive. Share resources, encourage others, challenge outdated ideas, and stand up for evidence-based, practical solutions. Every time you support someone else, you multiply your own progress.

From us to you, thank you for trusting, for letting us be part of your experience, and for bringing your own wisdom and questions to this process. We believe in your potential more than any expert plan or influencer could. We're excited to see the ripple effect of your choices, not just in your life, but in every circle you touch.

Here's to your wellness. It's messy, beautiful, evolving, and uniquely yours. Keep building, keep connecting, and keep recognizing your progress. The future is brighter because you're choosing to shape it, one step at a time.

BIBLIOGRAPHY

Ademusoyo. 2025. "How to Stay Motivated During Tough Times." *Ademusoyo* (blog). March 27, 2025. https://ademusoyo.com/blog/building-resilience-and-maintain-moti vation-in-tough-times/.

Al-Mamun, Firoj, Mohammed A. Mamun, Mark Mohan Kaggwa, Mahfuza Mubarak, Md Shakhaoat Hossain, Moneerah Mohammad ALmerab, Mohammad Muhit, David Gozal, Mark D. Griffiths, and Md Tajuddin Sikder. 2025. "The Prevalence of Homophobia: A Systematic Review and Meta-Analysis." *Psychiatry Research* 349 (July). https://doi.org/10.1016/j.psychres.2025.116521.

American Hospital Association. 2007. "Focus on Wellness." https://www.aha.org/ system/files/content/00-10/071204_H4L_FocusonWellness.pdf.

Anxiety NZ. n.d. "Name It to Tame It." Accessed July 5, 2025. https://anxiety.org.nz/ resources/name-it-to-tame-it.

Appleton, Jeremy. 2018. "The Gut-Brain Axis: Influence of Microbiota on Mood and Mental Health." NIH. August 2018. https://pmc.ncbi.nlm.nih.gov/arti cles/PMC6469458/.

Applied Behavioral Holistic Health. n.d. "Resilience in Action: How to Bounce Back From Setbacks." *Applied Behavioral Holistic Health* (blog). Accessed July 1, 2025. https://abholistic.com/resilience-in-action-how-to-bounce-back-from-setbacks/.

Association of Nature and Forest Therapy. n.d. "Scientific Review: The Benefits of Forest Bathing." Association of Nature and Forest Therapy (ANFT). Accessed July 5, 2025. https://anft.earth/research/.

Berman, Robby. 2022. "Having a Sense of Purpose May Help You Live Longer, Research Shows." Medical News Today. November 21, 2022. https://www.medicalnewstoday. com/articles/longevity-having-a-purpose-may-help-you-live-longer-healthier.

Better Health Channel. 2024. "Antioxidants." May 3, 2024. https://www.betterhealth. vic.gov.au/health/healthyliving/antioxidants.

Better Help. 2025. "Benefits of Laughter for Your Physical & Mental Health." January 14, 2025. https://www.betterhelp.com/advice/happiness/the-benefits-of-laughter-what- can-laughing-do-for-your-physical-and-mental-health/.

Brown, Daniel K., Jo L. Barton, and Valerie F. Gladwell. 2013. "Viewing Nature Scenes Positively Affects Recovery of Autonomic Function Following Acute-Mental Stress." *Environmental Science & Technology* 47 (11): 5562–69. https://doi.org/10.1021/ es305019p.

Calm. 2024. "5-4-3-2-1 Grounding: How to Use This Simple Technique for Coping with Anxiety." *Calm Blog* (blog). September 12, 2024. https://www.calm.com/blog/5-4-3- 2-1-a-simple-exercise-to-calm-the-mind.

Caruso, Catherine. 2023. "A New Field of Neuroscience Aims to Map Connections in the Brain." Harvard. January 19, 2023. https://hms.harvard.edu/news/new-field- neuroscience-aims-map-connections-brain.

Center for Mindful Psychotherapy. 2023. "15 Types of Healthy Boundaries and How to

Communicate Them." Mindful Center. June 15, 2023. https://mindfulcenter.org/15-types-of-healthy-boundaries-and-how-to-communicate-them/.

Cherry, Kendra. 2024a. "What Is the Fight-or-Flight Response?" Verywell Mind. June 17, 2024. https://www.verywellmind.com/what-is-the-fight-or-flight-response-2795194.

Cherry, Kendra. 2024b. "How Neuroplasticity Works." Verywell Mind. May 17, 2024. https://www.verywellmind.com/what-is-brain-plasticity-2794886.

Clear, James. 2013. "How to Stop Procrastinating by Using the '2-Minute Rule.'" Medium. May 27, 2013. https://medium.com/@jamesclear/how-to-stop-procrastinating-by-using-the-2-minute-rule-9f271b3ecf56.

Cleveland Clinic. 2022a. "Vagus Nerve." January 11, 2022. https://my.clevelandclinic.org/health/body/22279-vagus-nerve.

. 2022b. "Neurotransmitters." March 14, 2022. https://my.clevelandclinic.org/health/articles/22513-neurotransmitters.

. 2022c. "Malnutrition." May 4, 2022. https://my.clevelandclinic.org/health/diseases/22987-malnutrition.

. 2024a. "Limbic System." April 6, 2024. https://my.clevelandclinic.org/health/body/limbic-system.

. 2024b. "Everything You Need to Know About Habit Stacking for Self-Improvement." June 18, 2024. https://health.clevelandclinic.org/habit-stacking.

Coleman Collins, Sherry. 2025. "Scrolling for Health: The Risks Behind Viral Nutrition Fads." Eat Right. May 16, 2025. https://www.eatright.org/health/wellness/diet-trends/scrolling-for-health.

CompassAI. 2025. "Why Celebrating Small Wins Boosts Motivation." *Upskillist* (blog). January 31, 2025. https://www.upskillist.com/blog/why-celebrating-small-wins-boosts-motivation/.

Corliss, Julie. n.d. "Six Relaxation Techniques to Reduce Stress." Harvard Health. Accessed July 16, 2025. https://www.health.harvard.edu/mind-and-mood/six-relaxation-techniques-to-reduce-stress.

Covenant Health. 2024. "Is Sleep Debt Real? What to Know About Sleep Deprivation." October 31, 2024. https://www.covenanthealth.com/blog/is-sleep-debt-real/.

Cronkleton, Emily. 2022. "Hit a Workout Plateau? Here's How to Get Through It." Healthline. April 29, 2022. https://www.healthline.com/nutrition/workout-plateau.

Descourouez, Mary Grace. 2024. "What Excessive Screen Time Does to the Adult Brain." Lifestyle Medicine. May 30, 2024. https://longevity.stanford.edu/lifestyle/2024/05/30/what-excessive-screen-time-does-to-the-adult-brain/.

Donovan, Dade W. n.d. "Minimum Viable Exercise Plan: Get Moving and Improve Your Health." Drdade. Accessed July 1, 2025. https://www.drdade.com/minimum-viable-exercise-plan-get-moving-and-improve-your-health/.

EBSCO. n.d. "Cognitive Reframing." EBSCO Information Services, Inc. Accessed July 5, 2025. https://www.ebsco.com/research-starters/psychology/cognitive-reframing.

Espinosa-Salas, Santiago, and Mauricio Gonzalez-Arias. 2023. *Nutrition: Micronutrient Intake, Imbalances, and Interventions*. Internet. StatPearls Publishing. https://www.ncbi.nlm.nih.gov/books/NBK597352/.

Farnam Street. n.d. "Carol Dweck: A Summary of Growth and Fixed Mindsets." Accessed June 30, 2025. https://fs.blog/carol-dweck-mindset/.

Fischer, Kristen. 2024. "Grounding: Techniques and Benefits." WebMD. May 3, 2024. https://www.webmd.com/balance/grounding-benefits.

FitOn. n.d. "FitOn." Accessed July 1, 2025. https://app.fitonapp.com/for-you.

Fletcher, Jenna. 2024. "How to Use 4-7-8 Breathing for Anxiety." August 21, 2024. https://www.medicalnewstoday.com/articles/324417.

Gaines, Jeffrey. 2020. "The Philosophy of Ikigai: 3 Examples About Finding Purpose." Positive Psychology. November 17, 2020. https://positivepsychology.com/ikigai/.

Gilbert, Kylie. 2024. "How to Practice Alternate Nostril Breathing to Find Calm and Boost Focus from Anywhere." *Peloton* (blog). December 13, 2024. https://www.onepeloton.com/blog/alternate-nostril-breathing.

Glenn, Jason. 2020. "Night Shift Workers: How to Sleep on Days Off." HealthShift. July 24, 2020. https://healthshift.blog/night-shift-workers-how-to-sleep-on-days-off/.

Gerretsen, Isabelle. 2024. "Why Power Naps Might Be Good for Our Health." BBC Future. January 29, 2024. https://www.bbc.co.uk/future/article/20240126-why-power-naps-might-be-good-for-our-health.

Guinness, Harry. 2024. "The 5 Best Habit Tracker Apps." Zapier. July 10, 2024. https://zapier.com/blog/best-habit-tracker-app/.

Hamilton, David R. 2012. "Visualizing the Perfect Performance." Dr David R. Hamilton. September 12, 2012. https://drdavidhamilton.com/visualizing-the-perfect-performance/.

Han, Yimin, Boya Wang, Han Gao, Chengwei He, Rongxuan Hua, Chen Liang, Sitian Zhang, Ying Wang, Shuzi Xin, and Jingdong Xu. 2022. "Vagus Nerve and Underlying Impact on the Gut Microbiota-Brain Axis in Behavior and Neurodegenerative Diseases." *Journal of Inflammation Research*, November, 6213–30. https://doi.org/10.2147/JIR.S384949.

Harvard Health Publishing. 2012. "How Stress Can Make Us Overeat." Harvard Health. January 3, 2012. https://www.health.harvard.edu/healthbeat/how-stress-can-make-us-overeat.

. 2023. "Probiotics May Help Boost Mood and Cognitive Function." Harvard Health. March 22, 2023. https://www.health.harvard.edu/mind-and-mood/probiotics-may-help-boost-mood-and-cognitive-function.

. 2024. "Understanding the Stress Response." Harvard Health. April 3, 2024. https://www.health.harvard.edu/staying-healthy/understanding-the-stress-response.

. n.d. "Six Relaxation Techniques to Reduce Stress." Harvard Health. Accessed June 28, 2025. https://www.health.harvard.edu/mind-and-mood/six-relaxation-techniques-to-reduce-stress.

Hinchman, Walter. 2019. "Good Fat vs. Bad Fat: What Are the Best Fats to Include in Your Diet?" Swolverine. December 15, 2019. https://swolverine.com/blogs/blog/good-fat-vs-bad-fat.

Indeed. 2025. "Types of Motivation to Achieve Career and Personal Goals." March 4, 2025. https://uk.indeed.com/career-advice/career-development/types-of-motivation.

Insights Psychology. 2025. "The Dark Side of Positivity: When Toxic Optimism Hurts More Than It Helps." January 28, 2025. https://insightspsychology.org/the-dark-side-of-toxic-positivity/.

Jarai, Maté. 2024. "Everything You Need to Know About Micronutrients." Zoe. April 24, 2024. https://zoe.com/learn/what-are-micronutrients.

Johns Hopkins Medicine. n.d. "Sleep/Wake Cycles." Accessed July 1, 2025. https://www.hopkinsmedicine.org/health/conditions-and-diseases/sleepwake-cycles.

Jones, Salene M. W. 2023. "Learning to Live in the Gray of Life." *Psychology Today*, January 2, 2023. https://www.psychologytoday.com/us/blog/all-about-cognitive-and-behavior-therapy/202210/understanding-and-overcoming-all-or-nothing.

Katella, Kathy. 2019. "Why Is Sitting So Bad for Us?" Yale Medicine. August 28, 2019. https://www.yalemedicine.org/news/sitting-health-risks.

Kiley, Taylor. 2025. "7 Health Benefits of a Standing Desk in 2024." BTOD.Com. January 8, 2025. https://www.btod.com/blog/health-benefits-standing-desk/.

Kluger, Jeffrey. 2023. "How Perfectionism Leads to Burnout—and What You Can Do About It." *TIME*, January 6, 2023. https://time.com/6244829/burnout-mental-health-perfectionism/.

Komoder. 2024. "What Is Progressive Muscle Relaxation: Discover Its Advantages." *Komoder* (blog). September 27, 2024. https://www.komoder.es/en/blog/progressive-muscle-relaxation.

Laderer, Ashley. 2024. "5 Vagus Nerve Exercises to Help You Chill Out." *Charlie Health* (blog). January 5, 2024. https://www.charliehealth.com/post/vagus-nerve-exercises.

Lewis, Sarah. 2024. "Prebiotics vs. Probiotics for Gut Health." Healthline. May 22, 2024. https://www.healthline.com/nutrition/probiotics-and-prebiotics.

Lomer, Irene. 2023. "10 Reasons to Practice Chair Yoga." Antara Yoga. December 4, 2023. https://www.antarayoga.nl/why-chair-yoga.

Lumen Learning. n.d. "Homeostasis and Feedback Loops." Accessed July 5, 2025. https://courses.lumenlearning.com/suny-ap1/chapter/homeostasis-and-feedback-loops/.

Luskin, Fred, and Lyndon Harris. 2025. "Twelve Steps to Self-Forgiveness." Greater Good. March 26, 2025. https://greatergood.berkeley.edu/article/item/twelve_steps_to_self_forgiveness.

Maguire, Larry G. 2024. "Fixed and Growth Mindset: Why Carol Dweck's Mindset Theory Matters in the Workplace." Human Performance. August 30, 2024. https://humanperformance.ie/fixed-and-growth-mindset/.

Maurer, Todd J. 2022. "Why Some People Grow from Setbacks and Others Don't." World Economic Forum. January 10, 2022. https://www.weforum.org/stories/2022/01/people-grow-from-setbacks-work-mental/.

McGarvie, Susan. 2025. "Emotional Regulation: 5 Evidence-Based Regulation Techniques." Positive Psychology. January 9, 2025. https://positivepsychology.com/emotion-regulation/.

McNally, Melanie. 2024. "From Small Steps to Big Wins: The Importance of Celebrating." *Psychology Today*, June 12, 2024. https://www.psychologytoday.com/us/blog/empower-your-mind/202406/from-small-steps-to-big-wins-the-importance-of-celebrating.

Mheidly, Nour, Nadine Y. Fares, Mohamad Y. Fares, and Jawad Fares. 2022. "Emerging Health Disparities During the COVID-19 Pandemic." *Avicenna Journal of Medicine* 13 (01): 60–64. https://doi.org/10.1055/s-0042-1759842.

Migala, Jessica. 2024. "Box Breathing Is Easy, Versatile, and Can Calm You Down in Only 16 Seconds." *Peloton the Output* (blog). May 1, 2024. https://www.onepeloton.com/blog/box-breathing-technique.

Mind Mics. 2023. "Breathwork to Connect Mind & Body." *Mind Mics* (blog). October 21, 2023. https://www.mindmics.com/blog/blog-post-mind-body-connection-rdnh8.

Mindful. 2025. "What Is Mindfulness?" May 15, 2025. https://www.mindful.org/what-is-mindfulness/.

Mohn, Elizabeth. 2024. "Cognitive Reframing." EBSCO. 2024. https://www.ebsco.com/research-starters/psychology/cognitive-reframing#

Moore, Catherine. 2019. "Positive Daily Affirmations: Is There Science Behind It?" Positive Psychology. March 4, 2019. https://positivepsychology.com/daily-affirmations/.

MU Health Care. 2024. "5 Ways to Stay Active at Work." Live Healthy. June 21, 2024. https://livehealthy.muhealth.org/stories/cant-ditch-desk-5-ways-stay-active-work.

National Heart, Lung, and Blood Institute. 2022. "Why Is Sleep Important?" NHLBI, NIH. March 24, 2022. https://www.nhlbi.nih.gov/health/sleep/why-sleep-important.

NIH. n.d. "Positive Emotions and Your Health." NIH News in Health. Accessed July 3, 2025. https://newsinhealth.nih.gov/2015/08/positive-emotions-your-health.

Nike Training Club. n.d. "Nike Training Club." Nike.Com. Accessed July 1, 2025. https://www.nike.com/ntc-app.

Nourkhalaj, Yasaman. 2024. "What Are Exercise Snacks and Why Are They Important?" Lifestyle Medicine. July 2, 2024. https://longevity.stanford.edu/lifestyle/2024/07/02/what-are-exercise-snacks-and-why-are-they-important/.

Osman, Vahid. 2024. "Calm vs. Headspace—Which Meditation App Is Better?" Halo Health. February 19, 2024. https://halomentalhealth.com/b/calm-vs-headspace.

Pattison Professional Counseling and Mediation Center. n.d. "Why Smaller Steps Are Better When Making Habit Changes." Accessed June 29, 2025. https://www.ppccfl.com/blog/why-smaller-steps-are-better-when-making-habit-changes/.

Perform. 2024. "How Top Athletes Leverage Imagery and Visualization." Tryperform. January 16, 2024. https://www.tryperform.com/post/the-champions-edge-how-top-athletes-use-visualization-to-win.

Pilat, Dan, Sekoul Krastev, and Kira Warje. n.d. "Why Is the News Always so Depressing?" The Decision Lab. Accessed July 3, 2025. https://thedecisionlab.com/biases/negativity-bias.

Pugle, Michelle. 2022. "Can Stress Cause Death?" Psych Central. June 30, 2022. https://psychcentral.com/stress/is-stress-the-number-one-killer.

Realized Worth. 2021. "Prove It! The Science Behind the Helper's High." *Realized Worth* (blog). March 17, 2021. https://www.realizedworth.com/2021/03/17/prove-it-the-science-behind-the-helpers-high/.

Reddit. n.d. "What Are Your Favourite Habit Stacking Habits." *Reddit*. Accessed July 1, 2025. https://www.reddit.com/r/productivity/comments/1dw91ca/what_are_your_favourite_habit_stacking_habits/.

Reid, Sheldon. 2024. "Journaling for Mental Health and Wellness." Help Guide. July 19, 2024. https://www.helpguide.org/mental-health/wellbeing/journaling-for-mental-health-and-wellness.

Santos, J. D. 2023. "How Visualization Amplifies Positive Thinking and Transforms

Lives." *Medium*, September 26, 2023. https://thereal-jdsantos.medium.com/how-visualization-amplifies-positive-thinking-and-transforms-lives-15c36dc3ea1d.

Sedano, Isabela. 2024. "71 Well-being Quotes for a Happy and Healthy Life." TRVST. November 8, 2024. https://www.trvst.world/mind-body/wellbeing-quotes/.

Seppala, Emma. 2014. "Connectedness & Health: The Science of Social Connection." Stanford Medicine. May 8, 2014. https://ccare.stanford.edu/uncategorized/connectedness-health-the-science-of-social-connection-infographic/.

———. 2024. "The Scientific Benefits of Self-Compassion." The Center for Compassion and Altruism Research and Education. May 8, 2024. https://ccare.stanford.edu/uncategorized/the-scientific-benefits-of-self-compassion-infographic/.

Smith, Karmen. 2023. "Exposure Therapy for Social Anxiety." Talkspace. September 22, 2023. https://www.talkspace.com/mental-health/conditions/articles/exposure-therapy-for-social-anxiety/.

Somanathan, Sudarshan. 2025. "How to Manage Anxiety with the Brain Dump Method." ClickUp. March 19, 2025. https://clickup.com/blog/brain-dump-method/.

St. James Rehabilitation & Healthcare Center. 2025. "How to Use Visualization Techniques for Faster Healing and Recovery." May 22, 2025. https://www.stjamesrehab.com/blog/how-to-use-visualization-techniques-for-faster-healing-and-recovery.

Stanley, Pablo. 2019. "Always Ask Why Five Times." *Medium*, April 1, 2019. https://thedesignteam.io/always-ask-why-five-times-452345856bde.

Streit, Lizzie. 2021. "What Are Macronutrients? All You Need to Know." Healthline. November 1, 2021. https://www.healthline.com/nutrition/what-are-macronutrients.

Suni, Eric. 2024. "Mastering Sleep Hygiene: Your Path to Quality Sleep." Sleep Foundation. March 4, 2024. https://www.sleepfoundation.org/sleep-hygiene.

The Healthy League. n.d. "Reliable Health Sources." Accessed June 29, 2025. https://thehealthyleague.com/reliable-sources/find-reliable-health-sources/.

The Jed Foundation. n.d. "Understanding Social Comparison on Social Media." Accessed June 30, 2025. https://jedfoundation.org/resource/understanding-social-comparison-on-social-media/.

The Nutrition Source. 2020. "Mindful Eating." September 2020. https://nutritionsource.hsph.harvard.edu/mindful-eating/.

The Sill. n.d. "The Benefits of Houseplants." Accessed July 5, 2025. https://www.thesill.com/blogs/care-miscellaneous/why-you-need-plants-in-your-life.

The University of North Carolina Chapel Hill. n.d. "Understanding Mental Health Triggers." Caps.Unc. Assessed July 1, 2025. https://caps.unc.edu/self-help/understanding-mental-health-triggers/.

Thompson, Sarah. 2025. "The Science of Micro-Goals: How Small Steps Outsmart Goal-Setting Anxiety." *Ahead* (blog). January 22, 2025. https://ahead-app.com/blog/anxiety/the-science-of-micro-goals-how-small-steps-outsmart-goal-setting-anxiety-20250122-025157.

Todd, Lindsey. 2021. "10 of the Healthiest Herbs and Spices and Their Health Benefits." June 30, 2021. https://www.medicalnewstoday.com/articles/healthy-herbs-and-spices.

Trainer O&O Coach. 2021. "Why Movement Is the Essence of Play." May 10, 2021. https://www.oandotrainercoach.com/why-movement-is-the-essence-of-play/.

Tumilaar, Sefren Geiner, Ari Hardianto, Hirofumi Dohi, and Dikdik Kurnia. 2024. "A Comprehensive Review of Free Radicals, Oxidative Stress, and Antioxidants: Overview, Clinical Applications, Global Perspectives, Future Directions, and Mechanisms of Antioxidant Activity of Flavonoid Compounds." *Journal of Chemistry* 2024 (1): 1–21. https://doi.org/10.1155/2024/5594386.

UCLA Health. 2021. "'Free Moving' Dance Has Healing Benefits for Mental Health." July 22, 2021. https://www.uclahealth.org/news/article/free-moving-dance-has-healing-benefits-for-people-with-mental-health-concerns.

———. 2025. "7 Health Benefits of Spending Time in Nature." May 14, 2025. https://www.uclahealth.org/news/article/7-health-benefits-spending-time-nature.

Unplugged. n.d. "Managing Social Media & Phone Use." *Our Kinda Family* (blog). Accessed July 3, 2025. https://ourkindafamily.com/managing-social-media-phone-use/.

Vasquez, Isabel. 2023. "Does Dehydration Cause Fatigue? Here's What a Dietitian Says." *EatingWell*, May 8, 2023. https://www.eatingwell.com/article/8045761/dehydration-and-fatigue/.

Vossenkemper, Tara. n.d. "How to Use I-Statements Effectively and Accurately." The Counseling Hub. Accessed July 6, 2025. https://thecounselinghub.com/news/mkniuct0phmijh51wz0qb4ksstgfpq.

Warley, Stephen. 2025. "What Is Self-Awareness?" Life Skills That Matter. January 19, 2025. https://www.lifeskillsthatmatter.com/blog/self-awareness.

Waters, Jamie. 2021. "Constant Craving: How Digital Media Turned Us All Into Dopamine Addicts." *The Guardian*, August 22, 2021. https://www.theguardian.com/global/2021/aug/22/how-digital-media-turned-us-all-into-dopamine-addicts-and-what-we-can-do-to-break-the-cycle.

Whole Family Living. 2025. "Best Apps to Help You Move More at Work." February 7, 2025. https://www.wholefamilyliving.com/apps-to-help-you-move-more-at-work/.

Willard, Christopher. 2022. "6 Ways to Practice Mindful Eating." Mindful. December 22, 2022. https://www.mindful.org/6-ways-practice-mindful-eating/.

World Health Organization. 2025. "Social Connection Linked to Improved Health and Reduced Risk of Early Death." June 30, 2025. https://www.who.int/news/item/30-06-2025-social-connection-linked-to-improved-heath-and-reduced-risk-of-early-death.

Yeager, David S., and Carol S. Dweck. 2020. "What Can Be Learned from Growth Mindset Controversies?" *American Psychologist* 75 (9): 1269–84. https://doi.org/10.1037/amp0000794.